FEEL LIKE

SH*T?

How to Stop BEING Fat

To Lucy,
In peace &
health :)
Theresa

Feel Like S**t?

At my largest, aged 37 and a size UK 22 — check out the triple chin action!

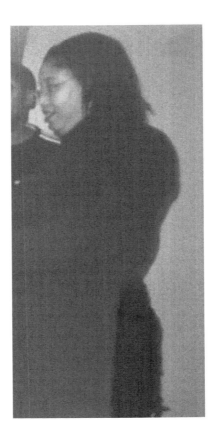

FEEL LIKE SH*T?

How to Stop BEING Fat

Theresa Fowler

Includes the
Sizedrop 42 Days to a New You
Food Plan

Feel Like S**t?

First published in the United Kingdom in 2013 by:
Theresa Fowler
Sizedrop Natural Weight Loss Solution
86-90 Paul Street, London EC2A 4NE
www.sizedrop.co.uk

Content copyright © Theresa Fowler, 2013
Front cover image copyright © Alejandro Dans Neergaard,
2013; back cover weighing scales image copyright © Luis Louro,
2013, both images under license from Shutterstock.com.

Back cover obesity free zone image
copyright © Andy Dean Photography;
author's image copyright © Pepe Ronnie @ visualbonds.co.uk.

Illustration on page 156 copyright © Theresa Fowler

B&W photographs copyright © Theresa Fowler, with the
exception of page 241, which is courtesy of *Black Beauty and
Hair* (www.blackbeautyandhair.com)

A CIP record of this book is available from the British Library.

Printed in the UK by CPI, tel: +44 (0)20 8688 8300

Cover design, layout and typesetting by Theresa Fowler
Edited by Donatella Montrone

ISBN 9781849143516

Acknowledgements

I would like to thank the following individuals, who without both their contributions and support, this book would not have been written:

Margo Marrone of The Organic Pharmacy, who opened my eyes to the toxic world we live in;

Ayurvedic goddess *Liliana Galvis of LilyPodYoga*, who at the start of my journey helped me find my core, and who continues to help me laugh so hard it hurts;

Jackie Ashdown for pushing me out of my comfort zone when I needed it, for believing in my abilities when I didn't and for becoming a trusted colleague;

Donatella Montrone, editor extraordinaire and long-time friend who's witnessed the ups-and-downs of this journey so far;

Nutritionist *Ian Marber* for his thoughts and time;

Richard Oakes for creating the space that allowed me to find the real me.

Contents

Introduction 9

Chapter 1: How You Got (and Stay) Fat 23

Chapter 2: Preying on Your Addiction 55

Chapter 3: Doctors' Orders 73

Chapter 4: Excuses and Choices 83

Chapter 5: Whole Foods for a Whole Body 93

Chapter 6: Exercise 125

Chapter 7: Accentuate the Positive 137

Chapter 8: Tap for Weight Release 155

Chapter 9: Action 165

Chapter 10: *Sizedrop 42 Days to a New You* 179

    Food Diary 185

    Daily Step Counter 191

    Days 8-27: No-Go Foods 192

    Days 8-27: Foods to Avoid 197

    Days 8-27: All You Can Eat 199

    Days 8-27: Menu Suggestions 204

Days 28-42: No-Go Foods 206

Days 28-42: Foods to Avoid 210

Days 28-42: All You Can Eat 213

Days 28-42: Menu Suggestions 219

Recipes: 220

Juices, Smoothies and Milks 220

Easy Lunches, Dinners and Sides 223

Sweet Treats 231

Best and Worst List 237

Natural Health Resources 239

Me: Before and After 241

Feel Like S**t?

It's time to step out of your comfort zone...

Introduction

I not only know what it's like to *FEEL* fat, I know what it's like to *BE* fat — to be fat, sick and unhappy.

I know what it feels like to have ill-fitting clothes filling the wardrobe. I know what it feels like to feel bloated and uncomfortable, yet still hungry all the time. I know what it feels like to be out of breath after walking up one flight of stairs. I know what it feels like to be secretly happy to

As a Thank You for reading this book, please visit www.feellikeshit.co.uk for your FREE BOOK BONUS

have flu, because it means you might lose a few pounds. I know what it feels like to hate having your picture taken, because you're always disgusted with the person looking back at you. I know what it feels like to cry yourself to sleep because of the pain caused by your thighs rubbing raw when you dared to wear a skirt without tights or leggings in the summer heat.

Increased portion sizes, sedentary lifestyles and the round-the-clock availability of 'convenience' food have all combined in recent decades to make us, here in the UK, the most overweight nation in Europe. Nearly a quarter of all adults and a fifth of children in the UK are now not just overweight, but obese (*Statistics on obesity, physical activity and diet: England, 2011*, The NHS Information Centre). In addition, a lack of nutritional education and/or basic cooking skills in schools; a lack of positive, healthy role models; a lack of adequate exercise for both children and adults; and a lack of personal responsibility about health have all contributed to the epidemic.

But the truth is that weight problems are caused by many factors, some of which vary from individual to individual.

We have become the most obese society ever to live on this planet. The fact that McDonald's, Coca-Cola and Cadburys were among the main sponsors of the London 2012 Olympics reeks of hypocrisy. The UK government's argument that working with the food industry, including McDonald's and Pepsi, is the best way to tackle the problem is also hypocritical, for allowing processed food manufacturers to self-regulate is dangerous.

The highlighting of the 'five a day' logo on some tinned foods high in sugar and salt is a good example. Another is the recent horsemeat disguised as beef scandal. Although the Food Standards Agency (FSA) claimed that the matter was not a public health issue and advised that the products were fit for human consumption, that doesn't take away from the fact that manufacturers and processors were complicit in supplying the tainted products, as well as misleading customers with labels that duped them into thinking otherwise.

Of course, if you choose to eat horsemeat, then I'm sure you didn't see it as a problem. However, if you routinely ate readymade lasagne thinking it was beef, but then discovered you had been eating horse instead, it becomes

11

an issue. The deception has meant that even those consumers who are more mindful of what they eat, because they read labels, were misled. The fundamental principle of food labelling is to make sure customers *are not* mislead by the label, which is exactly the opposite of what happened.

Another recent food scandal in the UK involved halal meat being supplied to Muslim prisoners, which was found to contain pork. Get into your head now that if you trust Big Food to provide everything that you eat, there will come a time when you will also fall prey to deception. Processed food manufacturers are fully complicit in the fact that they are misleading people through their marketing. This shows that corporate greed is taking precedence over the health of the people.

No wonder obesity rates are soaring.

We also live in a very toxic world, which is the antithesis of the natural, clean and healthy environment of the earth before industrialisation. The accumulation of toxins on a daily basis is the root cause of most disease, as well as obesity. Toxins are found in the air, earth and water, in the form of pesticides, heavy metals, industrial chemicals, electromagnetic radiation and pollution.

Toxins you may ingest on a daily basis are found in genetically modified foods, pesticides in conventional fruit and vegetables, antibiotics in meat and dairy products, soy, white flour, table salt, MSG (used as a flavour enhancer, and found in flavoured crisps and Chinese food) and yeast extract, microwave foods, refined white sugar, artificial sweeteners (aspartame), trans fat (including rapeseed/canola oil), caffeine, alcohol and prescription drugs.

And yes, the body does have the ability to detoxify itself through waste elimination and sweat — but only up to a point. In this modern world, the toxins we are bombarded with on a daily basis are far too many for our bodies to deal with.

Generally when toxic buildup in the body reaches a critical point, disease will manifest. But the complicity of the modern medical industry (Big Pharma) only treats the symptoms of disease — not the root causes. This perpetrator of the global 'sick care' system keeps people

As a Thank You for reading this book, please visit www.feellikeshit.co.uk for your FREE BOOK BONUS

ill and on medication. Big Pharma treats the symptoms and then any side effects, rather than educating people about disease prevention. Doctors are trained at medical schools that are funded by Big Pharma. After graduation, they write prescriptions for their patients for drugs that make people more sick and more fat.

Unfortunately, most doctors trained in conventional medicine are not in a position to help you get rid of your ailment or disease either. This is because their nutritional education is lacking and Big Pharma funds their education. So, doctors are trained to ply you with synthetic chemicals (prescription drugs) on some ruse that you'll get better. They do this because they get kickbacks from Big Pharma, which makes lots of money from it — billions. Current healthcare systems are not working for anyone except for those making money from it. All the while, the incidence of obesity diseases — Type 2 diabetes, coronary heart disease, cancer and so on — keep climbing at an alarming rate. What's so healthy about that?

If that wasn't enough to get you thinking, according to a study published by medical journal *BMJOpen* on 10

February 2012, if you do get sick and have to stay in hospital, then your chances of becoming malnourished can rise as high as 40%, and there is up to £13bn in associated healthcare costs.

And just so you know, conventional medicine doesn't prevent disease — lifestyle choices do.

We also live in a society that tends to stigmatise obesity, even though it's now becoming the new 'normal'. I understand this. For an overweight person, it can feel empowering to turn shame from that stigma into defiance; when society points its finger at you, blaming you and denying its own illness, there is a natural urge to send a message back to society with your middle finger. Which is why ad campaigns using 'real' overweight women cause such furore.

It's human nature to point the finger and pass judgment.

So, if you're overweight you can blame multinational fast food companies (Big Food) that aggressively market unhealthy (and pseudo 'healthy') foods. You can blame Big Pharma for aggressively marketing unnecessary over-the-counter painkillers and the rest. You can blame multinational 'diet' brands (Big Weight Loss) for their marketing propaganda. You can blame overeating or bingeing on a lack of willpower. You can blame your parents for feeding you poorly as a child. You can blame your busy, modern lifestyle, which has turned you into an addict of one kind or another — be it recreational and/or prescription drugs, cigarettes, alcohol, caffeine, junk food and/or sugar.

Of course, you can continue to make excuses and blame others about your weight forever, but who will that really help? You don't have to live in that matrix. I know you have the ability to pull yourself out of the system, because I was able to do it, for years never believing that I'd ever look and feel how I do now — at nearly 49 years of age. I grew up as The Fat Kid.

Throughout my teens and early adulthood, I kept piling on the pounds and eventually yo-yo'd my way to more than 16 stone at age 40. My GP told me I was genetically predisposed to being overweight. And by that time I had accepted my large size, trying not to let it bother me — on the outside. The inside was a different matter.

There did come a time when I was tired of being fat, but I was also very tired. I was tired of not being able to walk into any shop and buy what I liked in my size. I was tired of dreading the summer, because it would mean feeling uncomfortably hot and sweaty. I was desperately tired of my thighs rubbing, sometimes to the point where the skin was raw. I was tired of being humiliated in public by strangers who felt they had a right to shout abuse at me. I was tired of all this making me feel unhappy. I was tired of feeling tired all the time. I used to feel like shit.

Five years ago my father died an early death from pancreatic cancer, bought on by years as a Type 2 diabetic and related complications. His death was the slap in the face I needed to wake up to my reality. An early death was also exactly where I was headed. After my initial grief, I knew I had to do something about my situation. I had to stop *being* fat. So, I started researching alternative health and nutrition. I hired a personal trainer. I began to *invest in myself* instead of investing in processed food and weight-loss products.

Having previously lived a very toxic life and now living in good health to the best of my ability, my mission is to help as many people as I can by providing them with the most accurate information I know to help them heal themselves — and therefore others. So get this into your head now: to rid your body of the toxic fat that is basically killing you, a change of lifestyle is needed. Read that sentence again. *And again. And again* — until it sinks in.

I completely get that changing your lifestyle won't be easy. In fact, it has been the hardest thing I've ever done. But I'm no superhero, so I know that if I did it, then anyone else who puts their mind to it is also capable of the same. By far, it has been the most rewarding thing I have done — my life has changed in so many great ways I'd never before have thought conceivable!

For example, I now sleep through the night, having previously suffered with sleep apnea, and wake each morning feeling refreshed and ready for the day ahead. I used to suffer with excessive sweating, but now, apart from the odd hot flush, I only sweat in the sauna or when I exercise. I used to dread dragging my body up a flight of stairs, now I run. I used to feel down about myself, but now I love being me and I'm more optimistic about life.

So, if you're prepared that your positive change of lifestyle will also mean a positive change in your relationships, work and other aspects of your life, then the shocks won't be so hard. Of course, you may also probably resist changing your lifestyle.

Sometimes when I tell others that this is what's needed, the response I get is something along the lines of, "But there's no way I'm going to give up my daily coffee and/or wine and/or chocolate and/or whatever." Fair enough, I'll say. I'm not writing this to lecture you or tell you to do anything. What I can say is that the lifestyle you're leading now obviously isn't working for you. Or else you'd be doing something else — like not reading this book!

You have to get your brain really ready to lose the fat. 'Ready' being the key word here, because there is no magic pill that will instantly melt away years of excess weight off anyone's body. You did not become overweight overnight, so there is *no* way you'll be at your ideal weight tomorrow.

The great thing about life on this planet is that each day you get another chance at being or doing. It is you who

As a Thank You for reading this book, please visit www.feellikeshit.co.uk for your FREE BOOK BONUS

makes your choices. Yesterday's problems are in the past, while the present allows you to reinvent yourself. Basically, with the burning desire and will to succeed, you can transform yourself into the person you want and deserve to be.

I now realise that for years, I wasn't ready to lose my fat. For most of my adult life, I refused to believe that what I ate or drank had anything to do with me being obese. I counted my calories and stayed around my recommended daily allowance of 2,000 calories a day, so I knew it couldn't have been that. But what I ate was low-calorie, processed 'readymade' food products thinking, wrongly, that these so-called 'healthy options' were healthy. I believed the hype, like so many others out there.

So, what if you instead choose to truly live a healthier lifestyle? To completely change your lifestyle to a more positive one where you are happy? What if you were to learn from those who've taken the arduous and difficult — but ultimately brilliant, wonderful and life-affirming — journey from fat to health? What about turning shame into a commitment to greater wellbeing and happiness? What about refusing to beat yourself up with society's negative messages, and instead build a life full of joy, confidence and self-acceptance? What about the joy of having thighs that don't rub together? What about the pain in your feet/knees/lower back disappearing because you feel strong and healthy, not weak and in pain?

Only you have the power to take control of your health, no-one else is going to do it for you. In doing so, you'll have to accept and choose to live above the pervasiveness of Big Food, Big Pharma and Big Weight Loss — all with their Big Budgets for advertising and persuading us to use their products. Remember: their profits mean your ill health. Think about it — if everyone ate a healthy diet, these companies would be out of billions worth of business. These are the major outside risks to your health, but when you learn to stop buying from them and playing in their matrix, you'll start doing yourself an enormous favour. Your body will thank you for the rest of your life.

When   you're in good health, your thinking will be more positive, and you will feel more confident and happy. When I was fat, I had somehow convinced myself that I was happy, because I've always been very capable of having fun. Even as a 7-year-old during a lengthy hospital stay, I remember having fun. But I also remember the moment I began to feel happy, because at that point something switched in my brain, and it was then that I knew I had finally conquered My Old Fat Self. Now, I'm usually a 'Never Say Never' kind of gal, but I *know* that I will *never* be fat again. Not in this lifetime. I am better than she ever was. I actually feel sorry for her now for being so misinformed.

I am worth so much more than feeling like My Old Fat Self. She was never happy. She was full of physical pains. She hated the body she was in. I know which side of life I'd rather spend the rest of my days. Perhaps you feel the same?

Chapter 1:
How You Got (and Stay) Fat

Many factors affect weight loss, which makes the process of actually shedding fat far more complicated than the common belief that it's simply calories in and out. There's a lot more to sculpting a lean, fit body that you'll love than the amount of food you eat

As a Thank You for reading this book, please visit www.feellikeshit.co.uk for your FREE BOOK BONUS

or exercise performed. This is because the body produces different hormones in response to the different types of food and drink that you consume.

Think about where you get your food. Whether it's fresh fruits and vegetables, fast food or microwave pizza, the producers of these products have only one goal — to make money. Look at it this way: do you think you would make more money if your products were inedible after a few days or if they had a longer shelf life? Obviously, the longer the shelf life a product has, the easier it is to make money from it.

Food manufacturers also add preservatives, growth hormones, antibiotics, flavour enhancers (autolysed yeast extract and MSG), binders, fillers and other toxins, such as sugar, into the mix to help them boost their profits. Therefore, refined sugar, grains, refined vegetable oils and pasteurised dairy products are what has come to constitute the average western diet.

However, "glucose and fat intake have both been shown to induce inflammation, potentially through increases in oxidative stress".[1] So, all processed foods, refined carbohydrates and other modern food staples cause inflammation and promote fat.

Toxic Shock

Environmental toxins, such as pollution, nicotine, plastics, and chemicals in household, personal care products and pharmaceutical drugs, disrupt the regulation of the body's endocrine hormones, causing various health problems, including dangerous belly fat and diabetes. Toxins you may carry inside your gut could also include bacterial and yeast infections, chronic viral infections, as well as stress, anxiety or negative thinking.

Obesogens, which you've probably never even heard of, are foreign chemical compounds that disrupt the normal balance of your body fat metabolism, leading to weight gain. Sugars such as high-fructose corn syrup (HFCS), as well as nicotine, pesticides, pharmaceutical drugs, BPA plastics and some water supplies all contain obesogens. This is why detoxification of the body's fat cells is an important part of weight loss, but more on that later.

I know this will feel like unfortunate news for some, but alcohol is also a major toxin. It disrupts the delicate balance of nutrition, fluid and hormones needed to lose fat, and boosts cortisol, the hormone that breaks down muscle and makeshift belly fat. Binge drinking, even occasionally, increases the release of cortisol and slows down the metabolism, which makes it easier to gain more weight. And when you're drunk, you're more likely to reach for whatever junk food is your thing without being fully conscious of what you're doing. Even a daily large glass of wine will eventually make you fat if your hormones are out of whack and your cortisol levels are high through stress. I know, because I've been there.

Two years ago, I decided to give up drinking for three months to see if I could progress more in my physical fitness. After only a week off the booze, I felt better and stronger in my training sessions, so it encouraged me to keep going. At the end of three months, I bought a bottle of champagne to celebrate my success in staying off the booze and for losing another stone. After only one glass, I was truly pickled — prior to giving up the drink, it would have taken up to two bottles to have the same effect.

These days I'll have the odd glass of wine, champagne or beer every now and then, but I prefer feeling fantastic rather than bloated, weak and out of control. Plus, I save money on alcohol that wasn't making me feel great anyway. And I don't have hangovers anymore, which is all good in my book.

Setting the Stage

All of these toxins cause inflammation, and this is one of the main reasons why you can't lose weight. Dietary choices alone seem to be the most important factor involved in low-level chronic inflammation. The regular consumption of processed and synthetic chemically-laden foods leads to diet-induced inflammation, which sets the stage for various disease and illnesses.

The cells of fruit, vegetables, nuts and meat, when introduced into the digestive system, are converted into energy the body understands how to use. Processed wheat, sugar, HFCS and other industrial food are full of chemicals the body doesn't know how to process, which stress the liver and digestive organs and allow for toxins to build up in the cells, causing inflammation.

The processed foods that are eaten today have a higher carbohydrate density than anything man has consumed

27

on a regular basis during our evolution. This is why low-carbohydrate diets are generally effective in promoting weight loss. However, this isn't sustainable long-term and could even be a dangerous way to shed fat.

Fat Facts

There are two types of fat — subcutaneous and visceral. Subcutaneous fat is the kind of fat that sits underneath the skin and causes dimpling and the dreaded cellulite effect (which, by the way, is completely reversible if you follow a low-sugar diet... mine has virtually disappeared). Visceral fat is found in the abdominal area and can infiltrate your liver and other vital organs. It can also invade your muscle tissue and even has the ability to constrict your heart.

It is not unusually for thin people to have visceral fat because of poor dietary choices — have you ever heard the term 'skinny fat'?

Visceral fat is linked to everything from high blood pressure to Type 2 diabetes, heart disease and stroke. It has a very rich blood supply, as well as four times as many cortisol receptors as other body fat. Cortisol is secreted by your adrenal glands along with adrenaline. Both are stress hormones. A lack of sleep, or even too much, can also result in excess cortisol production.

Hormone Issues

The real danger happens when you are under chronic stress, because cortisol tends to store any unused fat released by the body's response to stress into the belly area. Plus, if your diet is high in any form of fructose, such as HFCS, you're more likely to suffer from chronic cell inflammation, which means you feel bloated most of the time. This is because fructose uses up a lot of energy in your body to process, so your cells become energy-depleted. As a result, they stop functioning normally and become inflamed. My body was in exactly the same state of distress not all that long ago.

Besides cortisol, insulin and leptin are two other hormones involved in weight gain. Leptin resistance is similar conceptually to insulin resistance. With insulin resistance, chronic elevated levels make your muscle and fat cells more resistant to the metabolism of glucose (sugar) in the bloodstream. With leptin resistance, chronic elevated levels decrease its sensitivity in the brain, so you'll tend to eat more than is needed. This also makes weight loss more difficult, because restricting food is something your body doesn't want to do.

HFCS also shuts down leptin production, which means your brain never gets the signal that you've eaten enough, so you don't feel full. And you keep eating and eating. And the manufacturers make more and more money. Are you getting the picture here?

With GH You Can Change

It's not all doom and gloom, though, because you can step out of the paradigm. For instance, there's good news on the hormone front — essentially, you can train your body to fight cortisol by producing more Human Growth Hormone, or GH. You also have the ability to reset your leptin and insulin levels.

GH is one of the most effective things in the world to offset cortisol and is produced by the pituitary gland. The big advantage of producing more GH is that it is your best weapon for fighting visceral fat. There are a variety of high-intensity physical training protocols you can use to make your body produce GH.

Two very effective ways I've used to help shed my visceral nightmare are the Tabata protocol[2] and Dr Mercola's Peak 8[3]. The best thing about using these techniques to help melt fat away for good is that they can be done whatever your fitness level with different types of cardio. And as an added bonus, they take no more than 20 minutes or so to do, so they can easily fit around any busy schedules.

Don't Trust The Industrial Process

Governmental healthy eating guidelines leave a lot to be desired. They are biased towards scandalous Big Food manufacturers that are out to make more money. "Government supports business, including the food business," argues nutritionist Ian Marber. However, I would like to add that these companies knowingly design and engineer processed food so that it is able to reside in warehouses for however long, be transported conveniently without much damage, end up on residing supermarket shelves until bought and 'taste good' to the end user. And again I ask, what's healthy about that?

As far as the supermarkets that sell the products are concerned, "They are businesses with shareholders and commercial interests, and whilst some people may not like it, they are charged with selling all food. They do promote health, but they also promote indulgence, treats, value, choice and low prices. In my experience, retailers do understand and accept that they have a responsibility, but it's not one specific to the nation's health, it's far wider than that," adds Marber.

I grew up in America in the 1970s, when TV dinners (with 'balanced' food groups displayed neatly in divided foil trays that were 'oh so space age'), convenience food and microwaves became all the rage. Introduced in 1958, Tang Instant Breakfast Drink had stagnant sales until an ad campaign using the Mercury and Apollo NASA space missions was used in the late '60s to boost business. Positioned as NASA's drink of choice, a nutritional and flavoursome breakfast 'substitute' for fresh orange juice, I clearly remember the ads for Tang on TV. My five-year-old self and younger brother nagged our parents to buy it. We idolised Neil Armstrong and the other astronauts, so if it was good enough for them....

The excitement of watching my mum pour the shocking orange liquid into glasses was hard to contain. However, two gulps in and I vomited all over myself. Even now, more than 40 years later, I can recall the synthetic chemical taste. I obviously didn't understand then that it was my natural instinct to expel the vile poison. The next morning it was back to orange juice.

After World War II, the US agricultural system was transformed by the use of industrial inputs such as fertiliser. This shift, combined with government subsidies for foods such as corn and soy, contributed to creating to a farming system that produces abundant quantities of cheap food.

This has stimulated the growth of an industry with a financial incentive to use corn and soy products (HFCS, hydrogenated oils, maltodextrin and so on) to produce processed foods. Supermarket shelves in the 1970s on both sides of the Atlantic became shopping paradises filled with colourful boxes and packages with 'sell by' dates that made us want them, because we had seen them being advertised on TV. Macaroni and cheese dinners, 'real' mayonnaise, wild blueberry muffin mix, strawberry frozen cheesecake, margarine, iced tea crystals, individually sliced processed cheese, non-dairy whipped cream... and on and on and on. What we were being sold, though, was a big lie.

Welcome to the world of Big Food.

Profit and Loss

There are many reasons why processed, ready-to-eat foods are attractive, among them being that in many households people must work (some in multiple jobs), which causes increased stress, and lower or stagnant wages that add pressure to household budgets. And as most food is shipped thousands of miles before it is eaten, the most profitable are those that ship well, have a longer shelf life, and can be 'branded'. Therefore, the modern food system is flooded with processed and packaged foods.

And unlike soy and corn, most fruit and vegetables are not subsidised, are more labour-intensive to grow and harvest, perish quickly, and are more difficult to brand, which makes them less profitable for food corporations. This means fruit and vegetables are not marketed, all the while processed foods are given more space on supermarket shelves.

Since the 1970s, the price of fruit and vegetables has also increased at a faster rate than inflation, making them even more expensive relative to processed food, which is why they can sometimes be more expensive than items such as soft drinks.

On the other hand, only 20% of all corn is consumed directly as food, and most of that is processed into junk; the remaining 80% is used for ethanol or animal feed, which fattens up the animals, but causes myriad health problems.

Fat is Good

Everything you think you know or have read about how much fat, and what kind, you should be eating is probably wrong. There is a great deal of misinformation around on the topic of fat. On top of this, most 'vegetable' oils on the market contain hydrogenated and 'trans' fat, which raises your bad (LDL) cholesterol levels and lowers your good (HDL) levels.

The misdirected war on saturated fats over the past 50 years has convinced millions of people worldwide that unsaturated vegetable oils are a healthy alternative.

However, not only do many vegetable oils turn rancid at a rapid rate, which means they become toxic when ingested, many also contain very high levels of omega-6 fatty acids, which when eaten apart from omega-3 fatty acids can cause heart disease and cancer.

This is what is known as trans fat.

Many vegetable oils may also be derived from GMOs (genetically modified organisms), including canola (rapeseed), soy, corn and cottonseed oils. These same oils, when hydrogenated, cause clogging of the arteries. And because they are also chemically altered to resist bacterial degradation, biscuits, cakes and cookies can last for months or years on the supermarket shelf, never seeming to go off. Avoiding these toxic oils for cooking and sticking instead to healthy fats, such as raw grass-fed butter, virgin coconut oil, extra virgin olive oil and hemp oil, will greatly improve your health and lower your risk of disease.

Fat should be an integral part of your diet, as long as you are choosing healthy options. The no- and low-fat diet myth is just that... a myth. On these types of diet, carbohydrate consumption is higher, as well as sugar intake, which leads to insulin resistance. Plus, if low-fat dieting really worked, there wouldn't be a worldwide obesity epidemic.

Messing with Mother Nature

Genetically modified organisms, or GMOs, which are also known as biotech foods, were brought to the commercial market from the laboratories of biotech behemoth Monsanto in 1994. They are different to natural foods on account of the fact that genes from other organic material, chemicals and pesticides are introduced into the DNA of the food on the proviso that it will grow with resistance to fungi, viruses and pests, therefore helping to combat world hunger.

Instead, malnutrition of the world population has gotten worse and GMOs have caused illness among the masses, including obesity.

According to *The Independent*, since as far back as 1999, the canteen at Monsanto's pharmaceuticals factory at High Wycombe, Buckinghamshire, only serves non-GMO foods. So if Monsanto's own staff won't eat this poison,

why is it fine for you to do so? And according to
investigative journalist Anthony Gucciardi:

*"After it came out that Monsanto's genetically
modified maize crop was linked to tumours and
organ damage in rats, the EU food safety agency
immediately went up in arms in an attempt to
find a chink in the armour of the scientific
research – as expected. After all, WikiLeaks has
revealed that Monsanto literally has enough
political pull to have major United States
politicians threaten 'military-style' trade wars
against nations that reject GMOs.*

*"One thing that went truly above and beyond the
call of political corruption, however, is the
agency's call to stop studying GMOs as they are
perfectly 'safe' and 'require no study'. A call that
obviously states 'please stop questioning GMOs
and revealing their true effects to the world'.*

*"After all, the study that linked GMO
consumption to premature death in both male and
female rats thanks to tumour development and*

38

organ failure garnered the most attention of any study performed on GMOs in the past. It generated massive awareness. The kind of awareness that profit-driven biotech corporations such as Monsanto simply do not like. The kind of awareness that could affect bottom line profits.[4]

Other manufacturers (mainly from food imported from the US) that use GMOs include (are you ready to clear out your cupboards?): Kellogg's (yes, those innocuous Corn Flakes, Rice Krispies and Pop Tarts), Nestlé, Kraft (Oreo biscuits), Cadbury (so that's no more Dairy Milk or Fruit & Nut for you if you care about your health), Hellman's mayonnaise, KTC cooking oil, Pride cooking oil, Hershey's Nutrageous, and OSEM sesame crackers.

Here in the UK, most GM crops being grown are experimental, and not commercial — currently. At the end of 2012, the Environment Secretary Owen Paterson announced his backing for the introduction of GM food production in the UK. GM crops grown at present include potatoes, rapeseed, corn and beets. In addition, a 2007 report by the UK's Soil Association, the organic food certification body, found that around 60% of the corn and

30% of the soya fed to cows and pigs in the UK was genetically modified.

The two other GM crops fed to animals are rapeseed and cottonseed, so even if you avoid GMOs in food products, you may be ingesting them unwittingly from the conventional meat you buy from the supermarket.

Even organic products containing soy have been shown to have been contaminated with GMOs.[5] Either way, it is impossible to live in true health if you regularly consume any of these poisonous products.

The Wheat Problem

Each year, more and more people experience discomfort after eating wheat or products containing it. This is because the wheat that's so readily available now is not the same type of wheat that was eaten 100 years ago.

In the 1960s, agronomist Norman Borlaug pioneered the development of a high-yield dwarf variety of wheat that refined already existing wheat strains. In 1970, he received the Nobel Peace Prize for introducing the dwarf wheat and modern agriculture to developing countries.

Borlaug's high-yielding cultivar, which had larger seed heads and thick, short stocks, was able to produce a lot of grain in a smaller space whilst being able to receive less sunlight than traditional wheat. However, it was also found that the dwarf wheat had lower mineral concentrations of zinc, magnesium, iron and copper, along with selenium. In addition, the commercial process of making bread uses refined, old and often rancid white flour, instead of freshly ground wheat.

Modern bread making also uses fast acting commercial yeast, instead of slowly fermenting with proven sourdough cultures as in traditional bread making. So, commercial white bread, pasta and other refined flour foods are fast and cheap to make and come in hundreds of varieties. But not only are most white flour products carcinogenic because they are also bleached and bromated by adding potassium, but any other vital nutrients are stripped away during that processing.

Avoid them, and all processed wheat products, during the **Sizedrop 42 Days to a New You** plan in order to give your body the chance to help heal itself. If you must give in to a bread craving (we're all human, so it happens),

41

essene or sprouted grain breads should help to satisfy any cravings. These are available in health food shops or you can make them yourself with a dehydrator, or an oven with the door open, and are easier to digest because the enzymes are left intact.

Also Watch Out For...

Monosodium glutamate (MSG), carrageenan and refined salts are chemicals that are often hidden in foods under deceptive names to 'enhance' the flavour of packaged food. MSG is a pervasive salt chemical linked to causing headaches, heart problems and brain damage.

MSG is also an excitotoxin, which stimulates the brain so that you eat uncontrollably. Scientists feed MSG to mice in order to study obesity, because it triples the amount of insulin the pancreas creates.[6] Up to 80% of processed foods contains MSG in some form, mostly disguised as 'natural flavourings' (superduper frappino coffee, anyone?), yeast extract and hydrolysed vegetable protein.

Carrageenan, another chemical additive often hidden in 'natural' and organic foods such as nut milks, can cause gastrointestinal upset and colon cancer. And processed table salt, which is added to just about everything, lacks the trace minerals that are normally present in sea and earth salts. Therefore, table salt robs your body of these vital nutrients. High blood pressure, cardiovascular disease and stroke are just a few of the conditions that can result from a refined salt intake.

And Another Thing

Other toxins that play havoc with your metabolism aren't so easy to avoid — polychlorinated biphenyls (PCBs) and dioxins, for example. These pollutants are byproducts of manufacturing and have been polluting our waterways for decades through landfill leaks and other sources, with the result that they've now entered the food supply through animal products. And despite being banned from water supplies many years ago, long-term consumption of PCBs from tap water may raise the risk of cancer and cause reproductive, immune and neurological problems.

Dioxins are a byproduct of incineration and other industrial processes at factories. They can build up in the fatty tissue of livestock that absorb this industrial pollution, so if you eat a high-fat diet from non-organic animal products, you are more likely to consume dioxins, which have been linked to cancer and developmental, endocrine and immune system disorders.

How can you avoid dioxins and PCBs? They only way to be completely sure is to buy wild or organic meats and dairy products, and remove the visible fat and skin from these meats before you cook them. I know that this process may seem over the top to some, who will consume commercial meat regardless.

I myself don't eat meat, but if I did, it is what I would do, and it is something you should keep in mind. Being more mindful of every mouthful you eat will make you more aware about what you are actually eating — meaning, will this food do me any good by eating it or will it give me uncomfortable symptoms?

Beauty Secrets

Did you know that cosmetics and personal care products are a huge source of endocrine-disrupting chemicals, which also wreak havoc with the balancing of your hormone levels. Beyond a well-established list of prohibited and restricted ingredients, manufacturers of personal care products *do not* need approval from any authority before launching a new product onto market. As a result, hundreds of questionable chemicals are included in the products that many of us rub into our skin each day (and your skin, your largest organ, can absorb up to 70% of what you put on it).

The most harmful ones you should definitely avoid are:

☹ **Formaldehyde:** *a preservative found in moisturisers, cleansers, shampoos, conditioners, body washes, eyeshadows and mascaras, as well as building materials and household products. It's harmful to the immune system, is a known carcinogen and is the main embalming chemical used to preserve dead bodies for burial.*

☹ **Parabens:** *are found in, but not limited to, shampoos, conditioners, body washes, tooth whiteners, toothpastes, facial cleansers, sunscreens and moisturisers. Parabens have estrogenic effects on the body, linking them to both breast and prostate cancers. In 2004, a study by the UK's School of Animal and Microbal Sciences at the University of Reading found parabens in* *samples of breast tumours; 18 out of 20 were found to have come from personal care products applied to the skin.[7]*

☹ **Triclosan:** *an antibacterial found in moisturisers, hand sanitisers, shampoos, conditioners, antiperspirants and toothpastes that can interfere with the metabolism of thyroid hormone and contribute to antibiotic resistance.*

☹ **Imidazolidinyl Urea:** *a formaldehyde-releasing preservative used in cosmetics and hair products. It is one of the most widely used preservative and is found in almost all water-based cosmetics, toiletries and pharmaceutical preparations. It is even often found in products labelled 'hypoallergenic', but can cause joint pain, fatigue, immune dysfunction, contact dermatitis, headaches, depression and eye damage, and is a known carcinogen.*

☹ **SLS:** *or sodium lauryl sulfate provides the foam in most commercial soaps, shampoos, detergents, toothpastes and other foaming products. It is* *cheap to produce, and mimics the effects of the oestrogen hormone. Because of this, it has been implicated in causing PMS, menopausal symptoms, a decrease of male fertility and an increase in female cancers (breast and ovarian), where oestrogen levels are known to be involved.*

And by the way, anything that says 'fragrance' or 'perfume', whether it's a household product, such as an air freshener, fabric softener or candle, or personal care product, including eau de toilettes and parfums, also contains toxic, hormone-disrupting ingredients.

Ever wonder why you sometimes feel overwhelmed when browsing the department store perfume counters?

For reasons only known to governments and manufacturers, perfumes, in general, are able to contain a multitude of poisonous chemical compounds, because the ingredients used to concoct the fragrances don't have to be disclosed. This means fragrances can be made up of any number from a stock base of 3,100 chemicals. Again, it's another example of how an industry is allowed to get away with selling you a poisonous product that is detrimental to your health.

In May 2010, the Campaign for Safe Cosmetics commissioned a study involving 17 brand name perfumes, colognes and body sprays for men and women. The study also found that, on average, up to 14 chemicals in each sample weren't even listed on the ingredients list.

In addition, these 'secret' chemicals had previously been shown to cause symptoms such as headaches and nausea, but were also linked to endocrine toxicity, abnormal foetal development, oestrogen disruption, sperm damage and even cancer.

This is because fragrance chemicals can be both inhaled and absorbed by the skin, so many of them end up in your body.

Stub It Out

Oh, and if you smoke, it goes without saying that you must stop in order to give your body the chance to get rid of the toxic fat you've accumulated. Besides the fact that you are quite literally burning your money away while you poison your entire body with toxic heavy metals and poisons (including formaldehyde, carbon monoxide and arsenic... yuk!), heavy smoking can also make you accumulate visceral fat in the abdominal area. This is because smoking increases insulin resistance, which, as you now know, is a precursor to visceral fat accumulation. This means while you may believe the common misconception that giving up smoking will cause you to gain weight, the opposite is true — smoking cigarettes will make you fat.[8]

And you know what? It's the same visceral fat that has already enveloped your vital organs, like your liver, kidneys and heart, and continues to release harmful molecules and hormones that will raise your blood pressure, stress levels and inflammation, and causes Type 2 diabetes, heart disease and some cancers further down the line.

Still fancy a drag?

Big Stink

By the way, I smoked heavily for 22 years — between 25 and 40 a day, although if I went on a night out or a session down the pub, that total could easily reach 60. I even had an ashtray at the side of my bed, because I lit up first thing after turning off the alarm and before getting out of bed. And the last thing I did before going to sleep was have a cigarette, which I now know is the reason why I never slept well.

I knew I was a heavy smoker and for a time I did enjoy it. I began smoking heavily when I was home for weeks at a time with chronic fatigue, out of boredom and frustration, and to numb the pain.

Smoking now makes me sick. I find it difficult to breathe when I'm confronted with the noxious fumes. When I made the decision to get healthy, it meant I had to stop drinking beer and wine. It meant I had to change my personal care products. It meant I had to stop putting chemicals on my scalp to relax my hair and accept my natural curls. So, it also meant I had to stop smoking, because that in itself was doing a lot of harm already.

At the time I knew smoking was bad for your lungs, but I had no clue it contributed to growing my visceral fat. It's no wonder my Dad died from pancreatic cancer after 30 years of living with Type 2 diabetes. He never exercised (I remember him riding his bike a handful of times when I was a kid). He smoked up to 40 a day. He didn't eat

50

whole foods. I knew that was also where I was heading, so I had to change it.

Leaving the System

With all this information, I've come to the conclusion that being overweight or obese are forms of self-abuse, whatever the underlying cause or reason, although the sufferer may not even be aware that they're abusing themselves.

I call it self-abuse because you're willingly choosing to allow your body to be abused by the system. Marber adds, "For some people who are obese, I reckon it could be [self-abuse]. Just like drinking too much or smoking."

Food manufacturers confuse us with marketing and the media would prefer us to be at war with our own bodies to help promote the latest fad. If they didn't have us hating our bodies so much, they wouldn't be making so much profit. So, if you are really serious about gaining your health back, you have got to pull yourself out of this matrix and take responsibility for your own body. Believe that now is the time to begin healing your body. As T Colin Campbell, PhD says in *The China Study,* "Both

[Type 2] diabetes and obesity are merely symptoms of poor health in general. They rarely exist in isolation of other diseases and often forecast deeper, more serious health problems."[9]

And you will have to put some effort in — just about everything you hear or think you know about your health hasn't been working to this point, which is why you're reading this, but know that the natural human default mode is health. It is where your body wants to be, so it should not be a struggle to get to where you want to be. It will take effort, yes, but no struggling. Plus, feeling better should be used as motivation to keep going, as T Colin Campbell adds, "impressive evidence now exists to show that advanced heart disease, relatively advanced cancers of certain types, diabetes and a few other degenerative diseases can be reversed by diet."[10]

Why is it that we have come to believe and trust in a system that basically does us harm? Or believe in the advertising of chemicals and processing, packaged in garish boxes, that have come to replace what nature provided for us? Only 100 years ago, there was no such thing as organic. Food was merely food, and it was what our bodies were designed to eat. The best advice I give to my clients when they are relearning how to eat is to begin by avoiding foods with health claims on the label. The next step is to begin avoiding foods that have labels altogether.

Think about what it would feel like if you could eat as much delicious food as you wanted without counting calories? What if you could feel self-love instead of self-loathing at the end of every meal? What if this new feeling of health and happiness lies just a few days away? Making small changes every day will give you the capacity to make the bigger ones needed to give you the permanent health and wellbeing you deserve. And only you have this power to heal yourself by taking the right actions.

But there's another big thing we need to talk about. It's another major reason why you're finding it hard to ditch the fat, and it's something you come across, all the time, every day. Sugar.

As a Thank You for reading this book, please visit www.feellikeshit.co.uk for your FREE BOOK BONUS

Footnotes:

[1] Steven E Shoelson, Laura Herrero and Afia Naaz, *Obesity, Inflammation and Insulin Resistance*, May 2007. Joslin Diabetes Center and Department of Medicine, Harvard Medical School, Boston, MA

[2] http://en.wikipedia.org/wiki/High-intensity_interval_training

[3] Dr Joseph Mercola, *Suck This "Magic Hormone" into Your Body and Transform Your Health*, 24 December 2010, www.mercola.com

[4] Anthony Gucciardi, *EU Food Safety Agency: Please Stop Performing GMO Research*, 30 November 2012, www.naturalsociety.com

[5] M Partridge and DJ Murphy, "Detection of genetically modified soya in a range of organic and health food products: Implications for the accurate labelling of foodstuffs derived from potential GM crops", *British Food Journal*, 2004

[6] John E Erb, *The Slow Poisoning of America*, 2003

[7] Rita Arditti, *Cosmetics, Parabens and Breast Cancer*, 6 September 2004, Organic Consumers Association

[8] Arnaud Chiolero, David Faeh, Fred Paccaud and Jacques Cornuz, "Consequences of smoking for body weight, body fat distribution, and insulin resistance", *American Journal of Clinical Nutrition*, April 2008, vol 87, no 4, 801-809

[9] T Colin Campbell, PhD and Thomas M Campbell II, *The China Study: Startling Implications for Diet, Weight Loss and Long-term Health*

[10] *Ibid*

Chapter 2:
Preying on Your Addiction

Foods that are high in fat and sugar are all too often perceived by consumers to taste great. Some scientists claim our preference for fats and sugars is explained by the fact that we adapted our tastes to the environment of our hunter and gatherer ancestors, where food was scarce — and where sugar and fat didn't exist together.

During times of scarcity, calorie-dense foods were more desirable and these were typically foods higher in either sugar or fat.

However, in the modern world, sugar and fat-rich processed foods are readily available, inexpensive and made to taste 'good' in laboratories behind the scenes, so that people are more likely to buy and eat them. Plus processed foods are generally high in *both* sugar and fat.

Eating disorders, which include both overeating and starvation, are behavioural as well as biological. It is about control as much as lack of control, with a mix of neurotransmitters, hormones, habitual behaviour and outside influences (media exposure and marketing) also coming into play. The brain chemicals that are turned on by drugs and alcohol are the same ones that go into overdrive when they encounter processed fats, sugars and carbs, which may go some way to explain why those who give up smoking or drinking find themselves addicted to sugary snacks.

Addictions can consume a person. But what makes eating addictions more difficult to manage than other addictions, such as alcohol or nicotine, is that the source cannot be eliminated. Every day we are constantly bombarded with images of processed foods on TV, on radio, on billboards, in magazines, on public transport, on the internet. So, anyone who's addicted to processed foods has that trigger confronted many times on a daily basis. And that's not including the colleague that baked a cake to share with everyone in the office (how could you possibly refuse such effort?).

Or the fact that you must also battle against the misinformation of 'healthy' packaged convenience foods.

Sugar, such as chocolate, sweets, cupcakes, ice cream, cake, cookies, fizzy drinks and cordials, makes you a processed food addict. Processed starches, such as white rice, pasta and bread, make you an addict. Salty snacks foods such as crisps and salted/flavoured nuts make you an addict. Fatty foods, such as burgers, bacon, chips, fries and pizza, make you an addict. All of these foods cause leptin resistance, which makes you crave more, and sets you up to further abuse your body.

With each mouthful of processed food you ingest, your body will react to it, hormonally and/or biochemically. Although you may think you feel fine, these poisons have a cumulative effect. The energy factories of your body's cells, its mitochondria, cannot process this junk, so your metabolism suffers. Although your tongue can be fooled and your brain addicted, your biochemistry cannot deal with this, so you'll gain weight and illness will eventually take hold. These days worldwide, most people eat mostly industrial, packaged, factory-made food products. For instance, are you aware that fast food fries are made of up to 20 ingredients and most of them aren't potato? Even a well-known 'diet shake' contains over 60% sugar, which is hardly going to make anyone lose extra pounds.

Your Daily Fix

Sugar itself is as addictive as cocaine, which means they have more in common than simply being white powders. In 1972, John Yudkin, a British physiologist, scientist and nutritionist, published *Pure, White and Deadly,* a book that examined the link between sugar and degenerative illnesses. Yudkin proved the consumption of sugar and refined sweeteners is closely associated with coronary heart disease and Type 2 diabetes.

In addition, eating sugar stimulates the area of your brain that produces dopamine, the neurotransmitter that regulates your pleasure response. When dopamine levels drop, you begin to feel low. This in turn makes you reach for more sugar to feel good again — just like cocaine.

Although you should be aware of all forms of sugar, fructose is the real bad boy, because it activates an enzyme known as fructokinase, which activates yet another enzyme that causes cells to accumulate fat. So, although you may religiously count your calories in and out, if fructose is involved anywhere in the mix, all of your efforts will be in vain. Food manufacturers also 'hide' sugar in many forms to fool you. For instance, high-fructose corn syrup (HFCS), linked to obesity, brain damage, low IQ, high blood pressure, cardiovascular disease and even mercury poisoning, is the evil twin of fructose. You should avoid all foods containing it, which can include breads, cereals, salad dressings and other seemingly innocuous foods like mayonnaise.

Industry Manipulation

You should also be aware that the refined corn industry, thinking it was clever and getting one over on 'consumers' when news of the dangers of HFCS began circulating, decided to change its name to 'corn sugar' and 'glucose-fructose syrup' in the UK. However, it's still the same poison — just under a different name to put you off the scent (remember, it's all about profit for these companies, not your health).

And if that wasn't bad enough, in 2010 a research team at Princeton University found that compared with rats with access to white sugar, those that consumed HFCS gained substantially more weight, even when taking in the same amount of calories. Not only that, but most of the weight was gained through abnormal increases in visceral fat — that dangerous, disease-causing belly fat I've been banging on about. You know, the fat that causes Type 2 diabetes and coronary heart disease. So, not only does HFCS cause you to eat more by shutting down leptin production, it also puts your health at risk.

According to medical researcher and leading authority on natural healing Dr David G Williams:

> *"Cancer cells thrive on sugars, particularly*
> *fructose. It has been demonstrated that cancer*

cells actually metabolise glucose and fructose differently from other cells. While cancer thrives on both, it uses fructose specifically to proliferate. It's no wonder that cancer has moved quickly up the list of killers in our society since we started adding high-fructose corn syrup to everything from sodas to bread.

"With such damning and irrefutable research, I still don't understand why it hasn't become standard practice to immediately put cancer patients on fructose-free diets to help disrupt cancer growth."[11]

And if you need more proof that HFCS is extremely dangerous to your health, a recent study published in the journal *Global Public Health* compared 43 countries, half of which had HFCS in their food supply.

Countries with citizens that consume none or very little HFCS include India, Ireland, Czech Republic, Austria, France and China. The highest HFCS consuming countries are the US (the greatest producer and consumer), Hungary, Slovakia and Canada.

The average American consumes 55lbs of HFCS per year. In the countries that consume greater amounts of HFCS, there is a 20% higher incidence of diabetes, compared with those countries with low consumption. The result was unchanged when the study controlled for possible factors such as body composition, carbohydrate consumption and population size:

> *"There were no significant differences in BMI or in other dietary variables, including caloric intake and total sugar intake, in those countries that use HFCS compared with those that do not. However, all indicators of diabetes were higher in countries that use HFCS as compared with those that do not."[12]*

So, the increasing popularity of HFCS worldwide should be considered a serious threat to health, because when eaten in excess, it causes negative metabolic effects including insulin resistance and weight gain from the accumulation of visceral fat (obesity).

Buyer Beware

Other sugars to steer clear of include corn syrup, rice syrup, cane sugar, glucose, beet sugar and even agave nectar, which has been hailed as a healthy sweetener but is refined (and sometimes mixed with other syrups) and anywhere from 50-90% fructose. There is also a large chance that the corn for the corn syrup and the beets used for the beet sugar will also be made from genetically modified produce if made in the US.

In addition, sugar causes inflammation in the body, which compromises cellular function. And it causes premature aging and stress (which has symptoms including unexplained exhaustion, sugar/salt cravings, moodiness and lethargy), candida and tooth decay.

Still think your daily chocolate or cupcake causes you no real harm?

No Need For Substitution

Artificial sweeteners are no better than sugar itself. Low-fat and low-calorie food and drink have the fat content taken out, so they include artificial sugars such as aspartame and HFCS to make up for taste. And although they are promoted to help you lose weight, there is much compelling evidence that shows sweeteners such as aspartame will actually cause you to gain weight. That's

63

right, aspartame — once hailed as a wonder chemical because it 'tastes' like sugar without the calories — actually makes you fatter, and adversely affects your blood glucose levels and insulin sensitivity.

The fact that aspartame is NOT a slimmer's best friend has been known by scientists for some time, but continues to be consumed in ridiculously high quantities through diet sodas. All because US FDA officials describe it as "one of the most thoroughly tested and studied food additives the agency has ever approved".

According to alternative health pioneer Dr Joseph Mercola, a study from 1986 that included almost 80,000 women found those who used artificial sweeteners, including aspartame, saccharin and sucralose, were significantly more likely than non-users to gain weight over time, regardless of initial weight.

I have first-hand experience of this. In my early 20s, I drank up to two litres of a popular diet cola containing aspartame every day. At the time, drinking water was boring to me, because I liked the buzzy feeling I got up my nose from drinking the cola. And because it was diet cola, it was only one calorie per bottle. I believed the myth that it was 'good for me'. I even got used to the aftertaste of the aspartame. That pattern continued for about four years until I was struck down with glandular fever at the age of 27, which was the beginning of five years of chronic fatigue.

During those years, I really piled on the stones, suffered tingling and pain in my arms and fingers, swollen ankles and knees, and got every cold or viral infection that went around the office (and would inevitably end up hanging round for weeks). In *How Sweet Is It? Cutting Through the Hype and Deception*[13], Craig Smith reports that aspartame "decomposes into formaldehyde, methyl alcohol, formic acid, diketopiperazine (which causes brain tumours) and other toxins".

When I think back to those diet cola days, it's no wonder I felt the way I did for so many years.

Neotame, a version of aspartame, is from 7,000 to 13,000 times sweeter than table sugar, and 30 to 60 times sweeter than aspartame. According to Dr Mercola, "Judging by the chemicals used in its manufacturing, it appears even more toxic than aspartame, although the proponents of neotame claim that increased toxicity is not a concern, because less of it is needed to achieve the desired effect."

Currently, neotame is not in wide use, although it is already approved for a large variety of food products because of its stability at high temperatures. And though it is chemically similar to aspartame, it has the addition of 3-dimethylbutyl, which is listed on the US Environmental Protection Agency's most hazardous chemicals list.

Sweet Repeat

Saccharin (marketed as Sweet'N Lo), which is much sweeter than sucrose but has a bitter or metallic aftertaste in high concentrations, became mired in controversy in 1977, when a study indicated that the substance might contribute to bladder cancer in rats. But in 2000, the chemical was officially removed from the US federal government's list of suspected carcinogens once scientists learned that rodents have high pH, high calcium and high protein levels in their urine, and this combines with saccharin to cause tumours.

As this does not happen in humans, there is no elevated bladder cancer risk, so it *appears* to be one of the safer artificial sweeteners. However, no-calorie sweeteners such as saccharin can cause the release of insulin, and hence weight gain, because of their super sweet taste. Saccharin is sweeter than sucrose (although it has a bitter aftertaste), which causes more cravings, and the cycle repeats over and over again. So, despite its lack of calories, saccharin still contributes to Type 2 diabetes and obesity.

Lethal Carbon

Sucralose alters the microflora in the intestine and "exerts numerous adverse effects", according to a Duke University study, including an elevation of liver enzymes, which negatively affects the bioavailability of certain nutrients. Sucralose is also an organochloride compound, or chlorocarbon.

In 2005, Dr James Bowen MD, a biochemist and survivor of aspartame poisoning, warned in *The Lethal Science of Splenda, a Poisonous Chlorocarbon* that "any chlorocarbons not directly excreted from the body intact can cause immense damage to the processes of human metabolism and, eventually, our internal organs. The liver is a detoxification organ that deals with ingested poisons. Chlorocarbons damage the hepatocytes, the liver's metabolic cells, and destroy them." And if that wasn't enough, more recent research suggests that if you are using no- and lo-calorie saccharin and aspartame by choosing 'diet' foods in an attempt to control your weight, then you are doing yourself serious harm, because they increase carbohydrate cravings and stimulate fat storage, especially visceral fat.

According to Dr Mercola:

> *"The belief that artificially sweetened foods and beverages will help you lose weight is a carefully orchestrated deception. So if you are still opting for 'diet' choices for this reason, you are being sorely misled. Ditto for diabetics, as recent research has shown aspartame also worsens insulin sensitivity...*

> *"The featured study, published in the January 2013 issue of the journal Appetite, was conducted by a Brazilian research team with the Faculty of*

Medicine of the Federal University do Rio Grande do Sul. Rats were fed plain yogurt sweetened with either aspartame, saccharin or sugar, plus their regular rat chow, for 12 weeks. Results showed that the addition of either saccharin or aspartame to yogurt resulted in increased weight gain compared with the addition of sucrose; however, total caloric intake was similar among groups...

"The reason for the similar calorie consumption between the groups was due to increased chow consumption by the rats given artificially sweetened yogurt... indicating that when your body gets a hit of sweet taste without the calories to go with it, it adversely affects your appetite control mechanisms, causing increased food cravings."[14]

Not So Sweet

Obviously, it would be completely implausible to say you'll never eat sugar again, because at some point you will eat the chocolate your best friend bought, or you'll join in and have the homemade cake at the office party. However, during the 12 weeks that you'll be on the

Sizedrop 42 Days to a New You plan, you will do your best to avoid any form of sugar or sugar substitute (aside from the fruit that you are allowed on the plan).

Besides, by cutting out the sugar, you'll be doing your body a world of good by giving your liver a good chance to rid itself of any built-up toxins. You'll also greatly reduce your chances of developing tooth decay and gum disease. You'll reduce the inflammation and bloating you want. And you'll increase your chances of feeling better with each day, looking younger with clearer skin and reducing stress. Good or good?

So, think you've got what it takes?

Footnotes:

[11]Craig Smith, Editor, *Alliance For Natural Health*, 8 February 2001

[12]Dr David G Williams, *Alternatives*, June 2010

[13]Michael I Goran, et al. "High fructose corn syrup and diabetes prevalence: A global perspective", *Journal of Global Health*, 28 November 2012

[14]Dr Joseph Mercola, *Artificial Sweeteners Cause Greater Weight Gain than Sugar, Yet Another Study Reveals*, 4 December 2012

Feel Like S**t?

Chapter 3:
Doctors' Orders

Because there's a lot of misinformation available about weight loss, most women fail to understand the difference between losing fat and water weight. Our bodies are made up of about 65% water, and when we first start losing weight when following a calorie-restricted diet, or starvation (we've all been there), we flush out large amounts of water, which in turn drops your weight.

If you continue to lose water for, say, a month, you'll look less bloated. However, your body will regain the water at the earliest opportunity. Plus, when you become dehydrated through water loss, you'll suffer from dry, flaky skin and lips, as well as lacklustre hair. You'll also lose any muscle tone you may have, which will make your body feel and look very flabby.

So, any weight loss that you may have achieved through starving yourself of proper nutrition — from either not eating or from severe calorie restriction — will reverse itself eventually. And when it does, you'll more than likely begin to eat more than you did before (it's that leptin thing again).

This is because the extra calories you eat will 'discover' that your body is in 'famine' mode as a consequence of its lowered metabolism. So, you'll store all those excess calories as fat, and before you know it, you've piled the weight back on. Sound familiar?

Unfortunately, your trusted doctor is probably not the best person to be advising you on dropping your weight either. In fact, nutrition is not something most GPs have the foggiest clue about. "That's not their role as a doctor. Their role is as a practitioner of medicine, and nutrition is not medicine. Some doctors do give nutrition advice — well meaning, but misguided and often amateur," says Ian Marber.

Nikhil Rao, a resident in psychiatry, adds:

> "We don't learn the basics of healthy nutrition. We don't learn about cardiovascular and musculoskeletal adaptations and responses to exercise. We don't learn about how insulin facilitates the utilisation of protein and creatine [an organic acid that helps to supply energy to all cells]. We don't even learn what all of those muscles in the body actually do... most doctors aren't even aware of the concept of high-intensity interval training, let alone how much more effective it is than steady state cardio.
> "And yet doctors think that their opinions on eating right and exercising actually matter. I

honestly don't know whether to laugh or cry about it. All of those years of school, and everything I know about exercise and nutrition I had to teach myself... And most of my colleagues don't see why I make such a big deal about it. There's nothing else to call it but pathetic."[15]

However, most people wouldn't think _____ about questioning their doctor's advice, even if they recommend they consume poisonous margarine because it's 'low in saturated fat and good for your cholesterol'.

NHS stands for National Health Service, but I don't see what's healthy about a system that dispenses pharmaceutical drugs to mask the symptoms of conditions that will eventually need treating when they turn into chronic diseases. Marber adds, "The NHS is there to fix, not prevent. Prevention may make sense, but I reckon it's more costly."

Meal Management

And just think about your GP, who more than likely doesn't have a clue about nutrition. Are they fit and healthy enough to be giving you advice about what you should be eating — especially if they say margarine is good for you? With that being the case, it's up to you to get your own health back on track. Empowering yourself with the right information will see you reach the goal you so deserve.

So, you know now that the only real way to lose weight properly, and to keep it off, is to manage your eating. This means up to six small meals throughout the day, rather than three main meals, which works because it increases your metabolism by helping to keep your blood sugar levels constant, making it possible to lose weight much more easily.

I know that may seem contradictory at first glance — that you should eat more often to lose weight. However, remember that everything you've ever been told before about weight loss hasn't worked. That's because of all the confused noise about fad diets, acai berry capsules or slimming teas. So, isn't it time to embrace the truth and give the *Sizedrop 42 Days to a New You* plan a go?

Now that you know the Big Food, Big Pharma and Big Weight Loss industries do everything they can to boost

As a Thank You for reading this book, please visit www.feellikeshit.co.uk for your FREE BOOK BONUS

their own profits, which in turn sabotages your health, isn't it time you do something about it to take back control? This is all about changing your current relationship with food.

In Your Own Hands

You are entering into a new chapter of your life that involves living a healthy lifestyle, and that means acknowledging that you must stop eating (and drinking) the way you do now. Because if what you have been doing was working for you, then you wouldn't be reading this in the first place.

So, where's the good news? Well, after following the *Sizedrop 42 Days to a New You* plan, you'll definitely find it much easier to adhere to a new, healthy way of living. For instance, you now know the evidence is quite clear that chronically raising your blood glucose through the consumption of refined grains and sugars will increase your insulin resistance, which in turn will increase insulin and leptin resistance. And avoiding insulin and leptin resistance is perhaps the most important factor to consider if you want optimal health, longevity and the body of your dreams.

With that said, the degree to which you choose to reduce carbohydrates is, ultimately, up to you. Just like clothing, what works for some won't necessarily work the same way for others. The main point is to become aware that when you eat sugar and refined grains and carbohydrates (not vegetables), it will promote insulin resistance to some degree or other, depending on the amount you consume.

What you must start doing is paying attention and being conscious about what, when and how you eat, as well as how it makes you feel. Problem is, there's more to it than just reaching for what you think tastes good.

Habitual Behaviours

For instance, have you ever really considered why you eat what you do? Or have you never thought about it?

Do you just mindlessly choose the cheapest products at the supermarket? Or do you overeat as a mechanism to cope with fear, loneliness or other negative emotions?
Do you indulge in sweet or fatty foods to reward yourself after a long, hard day or when you're 'treating' yourself

on a job done good? Do you overeat because you want to be socially acceptable? Do you indulge at parties so as not to offend the host? When you're out with friends, do you feel the need to drink just to fit in?

You must become more mindful, sitting down to eat, without distraction (turn off the mobile, TV, radio; put down the book, magazine). You must savour and chew every single mouthful, becoming aware of how it feels as it travels to your stomach. You should become aware of your digestive process and how it makes you feel when you eat such amazing, nutritious food.

Psychology shows us that our behaviours can change by refocusing our thought patterns — and all the while you are losing weight on the *Sizedrop 42 Days to a New You* plan, you will also be eating very well, so it's a double bonus. And all without ever experiencing hunger! This is not a fantasy.

A Big Food weight-loss program that requires you to starve yourself of calories and nutrients to lose the weight (and consume HFCS and aspartame) is restrictive and eventually comes at a cost in terms of your health in the long term.

With knowledge, and with some practice and cognitive conditioning, bad (or in my case, <u>appalling</u>) eating habits can be overcome. You can work to eliminate the negative and increase the positive in your circle of influence quite easily. For example, I've already mentioned turning off the TV when eating.

Or is snacking your problem? In that case, you could turn to your favourite music and dance around the room as a healthy alternative. Better yet, get some fresh air and exercise by taking a walk around the block. Play an active game with your children or spouse. Or spend some time in a mindful meditation to end the day in peaceful reflection. You should also become more aware of what media you and your children are being exposed to; you do have control over this and you can use it to your advantage.

All these activities will help you tune in to your body. Learn to listen, as your body will give you feedback if what you are doing is right (or wrong) for you. Learn to listen to that feedback.

As a Thank You for reading this book, please visit www.feellikeshit.co.uk for your FREE BOOK BONUS

Footnotes:

[15]Nikhil Rao, *What Your Doc Doesn't Know About Weightlifting*, www.t-nation.com, 17 Apr 2009

Chapter 4:
Excuses and Choices

You now have the knowledge to take action on seeking out the most nutritious foods available to you. But what about the other excuses you may use as a deflection of your fat reality? How many times a day do your thoughts complain about your size?

How many times have you self-sabotaged a dieting effort by reaching for cake because you needed the sugar? How many times have you blamed others (such as parents or a partner) for your poor food choices?

To become that better version of yourself, you need to realise that it takes a conscious mind to make your own decisions, which include your food choices. It's time to ditch the excuses. This is now about establishing healthy habits. Emotions often trigger bad behaviours, like overeating. The key is to identify the things that are making you feel pressured, sad, angry or anxious. Once you have identified your emotional triggers, you can break the cycle and start taking back control of your bad eating habits. When you change your attitude, you change your life.

A key element of changing your attitude is reversing negative self-talk. It's this kind of useless negativity that holds you back, keeping you from being the best you that you can be. Now is the time to turn it around once and for all. I can't remember how many times I've heard women say that eating healthily is just too expensive. My response tends to be, 'So, the prospect of dying from a

84

horrid disease will actually save you money?' Another common excuse is, 'I don't have the time to exercise.' My [admittedly sarcastic] response is usually something along the lines of: 'Is that because you just had to find out what happened in last night's episode of *EastEnders*?'

Big Boned Bullshit

At a certain point in my fat existence, I was Queen of Excuses. For starters, I *believed* the family bullshit about being 'big boned', which I now know was utter nonsense. When asked by the school nurse why I hadn't lost any weight after a previous weigh-in (in the late 1970s, when few other children tipped the scales), I blamed my parents who didn't allow me to leave the dinner table until I had eaten everything on my plate.

At uni, when I was able to make my own food decisions for the first time, I started to gain weight in a big way (no pun intended). However, I blamed my expanding waist on what was being fed to us in the dorm cafeteria (not taking into account the midnight pancakes my friends and I would feast on at the local diner, and the fact that I used to dodge the cafeteria salad bar for the much 'tastier' options).

When in my early 20s, having learned about starvation dieting and using laxatives from a former flatmate, I blamed the fact that I was still gaining weight on myself — well, surely there must have been something wrong with me! However, there was only something wrong with the bad choices that I was making at the time.

Smoking 60 cigarettes a day, guzzling two litres of diet cola, barely eating any fresh vegetables and getting drunk on lager and vodka slimline tonics were what was making me fat, but because I was having fun, I just didn't see it that way.

Yet that wasn't a sustainable way to live in the long term. I was merely existing and falling into a deeper sick hole. First, at age 27, came the glandular fever. This was then followed with five years of chronic fatigue. Next came the varying skin disorders (chronic verrucas, unidentified spontaneous rashes, non-healing sores).

Then came chronic bloating and constipation. And then the dizzy spells. And the unidentified shooting pains in my arms. And the high cholesterol. And a diagnosis of pre-diabetes.

It was only when my father died that I finally woke up to the fact that if I didn't have my health, then I really wasn't 'living' my life to its full potential. I don't want anyone to have to suffer with not feeling their best, like I did. And there is no reason why you should have to suffer such pain in order to get your own health back on track either.

Here are some more classic excuses you probably have used instead of taking action (remember, I've been in exactly the same position):

- 'I have a slow metabolism.'

- 'I can't afford the gym/a personal trainer.'

- 'I don't want to get too bulky, I've seen those female bodybuilders.'

- 'I don't want to get too thin.'

The key point here is that the excuses are not the issue and you need to look at the bigger picture. When you really want to do something, you'll find a way to do it.

As a Thank You for reading this book, please visit www.feellikeshit.co.uk for your FREE BOOK BONUS

And you won't care how long it takes. Otherwise, you'll make an excuse — and you may not even know you're doing it. Whatever reason or justification you come up with will seem perfectly reasonable at the time, so you'll rationalise it to yourself as just being a stumbling block, ('People die of hypothermia, so I'll wait until summer to start exercising'). You'll even explain it with plausible regret ('I really wanted to get started, but my partner's just not ready for me to become a strong, sexy, confident and energetic woman, so I just need to take care of my relationship first').

Please believe me when I say I get it. I *really* do. Countless people better qualified and experienced than me have studied this stuff in depth. Basically, though, what you're afraid of is failure, because you may have failed too many times in the past (did someone say Atkins, Dukan, maple syrup, South Beach, whatever?). If you're happy with this situation (although if you are reading this, you're probably not), then by all means carry on with your life the way it is. Again, I'm not here to tell you what to do, but don't be surprised when the disease diagnosis rears its ugly head — because it will. However, if you're at all motivated to stop making excuses, then now is the time to take action. If you want to feel better, stronger, healthier, fitter and at peace in your own skin, you must face the fact that now is the time to change. And although you'll be doing it in one goal at a time, the end result will be worth it.

Your first step towards your goal doesn't have to be big, but you must start somewhere now. And keep doing that thing. Just imagine how proud you'll feel about yourself in another week, month, year, five years....

Mistakes — I've Made A Few

The major problem with the average woman, like you, who is attempting to transform her body, is that she makes most, if not all, of the following bad choices:

- She skips breakfast (in a bid to reduce calories);
- She eats too many refined carbohydrates (white pasta, bread, cupcakes, and so on);
- She eats far too little good-quality protein;
- She thinks 'healthy' dietary fat means no fat;
- She's not supplementing her diet;
- She undereats in the first half of the day and overeats in the second half;

89

- She doesn't lift heavy enough weights (if at all) or do any other resistance training;
- She eats infrequently (meals too far apart or not enough);
- She eats her biggest meal at night; often a binge or 'out of control' meal (so she wakes up not hungry, skips breakfast and starts the cycle all over again).

These negative habits and patterns are what give women the disappointing results they end up achieving. It's why the radical celebrity-style transformations some truly expect will happen never come to fruition. Unfortunately, they have no idea how much work is really involved in achieving those results.

One of the UK's leading weight loss companies, which makes millions each year from its products and services, quietly acknowledges that as little as 6% of its customers experience lasting weight/fat loss. Why is this important? Because chances are, almost every woman at the gym (or Zumba class) is there because of some 'fat loss' promise, but without having all the facts. As a result, their expectations will never match reality.

The whole process of ditching fat is really simple — if you stick with it. And it's you who has to stick with it, because no-one else can do this for you. It's all about the *choices* you make. This doesn't mean there is a perfect way of doing it, just that you need to be aware of whether it is the better choice for you.

Everyone has a different body. Everyone has a different level of mindset. Everyone's motivation is different. But do know that everyone — including you — has the ability to change for the better. It won't happen overnight, or even within the first two weeks, but it will happen if you stick with it. Again, it is all about the *choices* you make. Yes, you will want to cry at times. Yes, you will feel that you're struggling and think nothing will ever get you out of the flabby skin you've found yourself in. But what you do then is stop, wipe away your tears, stand up tall — and keep moving towards your goal. *Because you can!*

Best Choices

For those of you who think you may struggle to get started, to keep going or just to see any progress at all, simply start by following at least one these four rules daily until they become part of your daily routine:

1. **Always eat breakfast.** Make it healthy by including a high-quality protein and at least one serving of vegetable or dark-skinned fruit.

2. **Drink filtered water.** Start with at least 2 litres and work your way up to 3 litres per day.

3. **Small and cold.** Make your last meal of the day smaller and colder by including a raw salad with it.

4. **Good-quality protein.** Start having protein (meat/fish/eggs/pulses) each lunchtime.

And then take it from there. Assuming you're now overweight and you perfect each of these steps, within six months I can guarantee you'll be much leaner. If one of the steps doesn't apply to you, then simply move on to the next one.

Chapter 5:
Whole Foods for a
Whole Body

Junk is defined in the dictionary as: "anything that is regarded as worthless, meaningless, or contemptible". Clearly, this is the antithesis of the definition for food. Therefore, to call something "junk food" is like saying, "I am healthy obese." So, in my eyes, there is no such thing as junk food. There is only whole food or packaged poison.

Using an analogy, think about your car. If you drove a car with a diesel engine, you would definitely think twice before you filled it up with unleaded petrol, or vice versa. Therefore, your body, being a finely tuned 'engine', needs to be filled with the correct fuel in order to run properly.

Being creatures of habit, we usually buy the same foods each trip to the supermarket, along with the odd 'special offer', without really thinking about it. Then, when it comes to eating, it's either shovelled in quickly without tasting it, or eaten on the run in a rush. So, when is the last time you really tasted the succulence of a juicy nectarine? Or savoured the sublime deliciousness of a blackberry off the vine?

Every bite of food you take should be savoured, just like you would wine at a wine tasting, because the more you immerse yourself in nutritious food, the more pleasure you'll feel in eating it, and the fuller you'll feel after your meal. With that in mind, let's see exactly what it will take to kick the bad habit of eating nutritionally inert processed food — your long-term goal. By investing your energy in yourself, it won't be long before you start to reveal the ecstatic being you really are.

Good or good?

The easy way to begin doing this is to create healthy eating habits. Start by incorporating more 'real' and less 'fake' foods into each meal, one step at a time. An achievable goal is to start the day with a healthy breakfast each morning if you're not already doing so. A nutritious breakfast will not only keep your body fuelled until lunchtime, but will also mean you won't reach for the biscuits at elevenses, because you won't be hungry. You're also more likely to be less irritable and more focused.

Healthy Habits

A great breakfast to start the day would be porridge made with almond milk or water, topped with a handful of fresh berries, yogurt and a dollop of honey. Or, alternatively, poached or boiled eggs with radish butter on rye toast (see recipe on page 225). Immerse yourself in your breakfast. Turn off the TV, radio or computer. Put your phone on silent so you won't be disturbed. Eating without any distractions will help you to savour the tastes, textures, smells and colours of what you are about to eat.

Another healthy habit to start is not skipping meals. Part of the enjoyment of eating real food is allowing yourself to get hungry enough to crave your next meal, but not so hungry that you're desperate to shovel any old crap into your mouth. And this state of being can be accomplished by making sure that you eat three moderate-sized meals at fairly regular times throughout the day, as well as having a mid-morning and mid-afternoon snack.

Some interesting and nutritious snack choices could be apple wedges with almond butter, or a few dried (unsulphured) apricots and a handful of unsalted pistachios. Or some hummous and oatcakes.

Mindful Mouthfuls

You know that Big Food adds bad fats, refined sugar and toxic salt to processed foods to mask the metallic taste of artificial preservatives, sweeteners and other chemical additives. And that your body doesn't understand these unnatural substances, so finds it hard to process.

Processed foods are also manufactured to dissolve quickly in your mouth, so that you eat faster and in greater quantities. Most of the time this leaves you feeling full, but not satisfied. So, you need to relearn to enjoy every mouthful of food, being mindful of each morsel and chewing it properly to get the enzymes in your saliva activated to begin the digestive process.

I've said it before and I'll say it again: your body's default mode is health. Therefore, the more nutritious the food you eat, the more your body will use it to its advantage, and the more you'll naturally enjoy it in the process. I see this automatic response as a win-win situation. Your body wants to eat real food. Not boxed, tinned or packeted processed chemical-laden readymeals. Once chemical preservatives are added or enzymes killed through heat treatment, food becomes toxic to the body.

The more you consider the vibrancy of the food you fuel your body with, the more you'll enjoy it automatically.

I know that initially it will be tough to skip the afternoon chocolate. This is why you have to take things one day at a time. One achievement at a time is what makes the bigger objective possible. You will be able to do this if you want your health and vitality enough, though. And gradually you will lose your taste for excessively sweet and salty foods as your palate adapts to the abundance of the new and nutritious flavours that await it.

Use this new motivation to try new foods. A good way to do this is by choosing something different that you've never had before each time you go to buy produce. If you're not sure how to use or cook your newfound vegetable or fruit, have a look on the internet for recipes — you're bound to find something that tickles your palate's fancy.

Taste Test

If you're still not convinced, you can test this for yourself: get hold of an organic strawberry. Examine its colour and aroma before you take your first bite, then give yourself a moment to savour its flavours. For a comparison, savour the taste of a strawberry-flavoured sweet or chew a strawberry-flavoured gum and take notice of what you taste. Is it succulent juiciness like the real strawberry, or chemically flavoured sweetness without any complexity?

You know that supermarket tomato sauce you like? It's one of those things you buy that you consider healthy enough. Well, the rule here is that if you must, or need, to buy packaged foods, only buy those containing five or fewer real ingredients. So, if your supermarket tomato sauce contains tomatoes, olive oil, salt, garlic and parmesan cheese, that's fine. However, anything out of a box, bottle or tin that contains preservatives such as sodium benzoate, thickeners like guar gum or artificial flavours, should be left on the supermarket shelf.

The same goes if it contains added sugars, hydrogenated fats or margarine. You'll also need to do the same for supermarket breads, breakfast cereals and pastas. If you're eating less processed foods and more whole foods, you'll be doing this anyway by avoiding most packaged products. But you should now be able to see that although you don't have to spend hours making your own tomato sauce, you'd be better off doing so. You also should look for products that contain the least amount of processed ingredients to ensure the best taste and quality. For example, it's impossible to experience the nutty chewiness of wholegrain brown rice if you choose to buy white rice. The same goes for wholewheat breads and pastas. And, of course, choose fresh produce, when possible, over tinned. Frozen fruits and vegetables are also preferable to tinned when fresh ones simply aren't available.

Meaty Issue

These days, when it comes to animal products, I eat sustainable fish, raw dairy and eggs, fruit, lots of vegetables, nuts and (mostly soaked) seeds. I supplement this with superfoods such as spirulina, chlorella, maca, cacao, chia and raw cow/goat whey, hemp and brown rice protein powders, as well as vitamins like C and D3. However, I don't eat poultry or red meat, and haven't done for 20 years.

As a kid I ate meat because, back in the day, I wasn't allowed to leave the dinner table without finishing my plate. However, I never really liked it — except for bacon.

When I was suffering from chronic fatigue, and bordering on obesity, becoming a vegetarian felt right to me, because I began to feel better than usual soon after giving up meat. Fast-forward just over 10 years later, and I learned through an intense session with homeopath Margo Marrone, founder of The Organic Pharmacy, that I had undigested beef in my intestines. Seeing as it had been more than a decade since I had ingested it, and it was still festering in my gut, I had enough evidence to prove to myself that meat just didn't agree with me. Saying that, I had only ever eaten conventionally raised and caged meat.

Don't get me wrong — I have no problem with meat eaters. In fact, being a 'never say never' kind of gal, I wouldn't rule out ever eating meat again myself, considering my constitution is now radically different to what it was then. What I do know, though, is that if I ever eat any meat, it will have to be sustainable, grass-fed, organic and reared by a responsible farmer. And I would never buy or eat meat from a supermarket unless it was organic. There are a couple of reasons why.

Main Course Horse?

First, when man began raising animals, cattle grazed on indigenous local grasses and shrubs, along with the goats and sheep. The meat of these animals was lean, nutritious and flavoursome.

However, after the Second World War and the mechanisation of farms, the strategy of farm production shifted to commercialism. So, the production of meat shifted to confining cattle in feedlots, where they are fed grain, corn and even sweets (that contain genetically modified HFCS, of course) as a way of lowering feed costs to provide even cheaper food to consumers, a practice that has been used for decades.

Today, most commercial cattle are confined indoors, fed unnatural diets of corn, grain and even their own meat (remember CJD?), as well as given hormones (in the US) and antibiotics that threaten the nation's health.[16] They are then churned out for slaughter in little more than a year. This 'efficient' process guarantees there will always be unhealthy, but cheap, meat available at the supermarket.

This same 'efficiency' process is used in the farming of corn and grain-fed fish. In addition, the grain and corn used is also most likely to be genetically modified.

Oh, and if the recent 'horsemeat disguised as beef' scandal hasn't put you off enough, just so you know, the UK Food Standards Agency has two classification guidelines on meat products — standard and economy. A standard beef burger must comprise a minimum of 62% beef, while a chicken, turkey or rabbit burger must contain a minimum 55% meat. A pork burger must contain at least 67% pig meat. Now for the really gross news: economy beef burgers only need to contain 47% beef, a chicken burger 41% chicken, and a pork burger 50% pig. This should have you thinking: "What's in the other 50-59%?" Think about it: if you have no idea what you are actually eating and how it affects your body, then you will always have a hard time losing weight.

You need to understand that.

Omega-3

Grain-fed beef and fish are also high in omega-6 fatty acids and have little or no omega-3. Too much omega-6 is another factor that triggers the body's inflammation response. And, as you now know, this is the type of chronic inflammation that often has no symptoms, so you'll feel 'healthy', even when you're carrying an excess of a couple of stone or more around your internal organs, your visceral fat — the fat that causes chronic illness.

You only need to look at beef consumption in Argentina to understand how eating grass-fed meat can be beneficial to the body. Although it is second in the world in per-capita for red meat consumption, at 58.2kg per head a year in 2010, the country enjoys lower numbers of deaths from heart disease, diabetes and cancer per 1,000 people. Plus the fact that Argentine grass-fed beef has been eaten for centuries.

Grass-fed meat has many benefits besides being more nutritious and raised without antibiotics. It has up to 10 times more beta-carotene, as well as three times more vitamin E and omega-3. And it is raised more humanely — and surely a happier animal will be more nutritious for you and taste better than an unhappy, stressed animal that lives in an unnatural concrete environment and is bred for slaughter.

Organic or Conventional?

This is a contentious subject. From my own personal experience, when I started eating organic vegetables and fruit, not only did I feel better, I also began to enjoy the flavours of the produce like I never did before. For example, cucumbers tasted of cucumbers, not crunchy water. Strawberries tasted of strawberry, not straw. Salad greens taste bitter and pungent, not like crunchy blandness. You get the picture.

But it's not just the taste that counts, because organic food is produced without the pesticides (also known as poison) associated with conventional food. This means you'll have a much better chance of losing weight and keeping it off, because you will be supplying your body with the cleanest fuel available to it.

And if you buy from your local farmers' markets, the cost of organic produce falls quite considerably, when compared with supermarket and specialty health food shops. Therefore, I find the cost argument that 'organic food is expensive' nonsense. It is very possible to eat mostly organic on a budget with a little bit of research and effort. Besides, would you rather spend a little more now on proper nutrition for your body, or pay a whole lot more later with a seriously sick, diabetic or cancerous body? Again, it's your choice to make the effort.

If you're not going to make the effort for yourself, you'll end up not moving forward toward your fat loss goal.

By no means am I saying that you have to shop organic at all times either, because sometimes it just won't be possible (when eating out with friends, for example). All I'm saying is that eating organic is preferable, since there are no toxic pesticides, hormones, antibiotics and residues in the food for your body to deal with. This will help your body to rid itself of the toxic buildup residing in your fat cells, which will allow your fat cells to shrink and your muscle tone to shine through.

As I said before, the produce at your local farmer's markets will also be of excellent quality. Or perhaps you're lucky enough to live near a farm or have access to a garden for growing your own.

As well, there may be times when you can only get hold of conventional produce, so washing and peeling of skins will be necessary. In which case, it is far better to eat conventional than resort to non-nutritional convenience food. Most studies find little difference between the mineral content of organic and conventional stuff. The biggest determinant of mineral density in food appears to be geographical location, because different regions have different soil compositions. Even members of the same vegetable variety from different parts of the country can have different levels of minerals depending on the soil.

However, it has been proven that organic crops have higher levels of magnesium, iron, vitamin C and phosphorus, with lower levels of nitrates because of the practices and systems used by organic farmers when tending to the soil, making the food more nutritious.

Green Party

And as far as vegetables are concerned, you want to make sure that you're eating your greens at every meal. Of course, lettuce is fine once in a while, but I'm talking real greens, such as spinach, dandelion greens, kale, watercress and bok choy. If you're unsure as to how to prepare them, you'll find tons of recipes online or in cookbooks.

It is impossible for the body to be nourished if you don't regularly absorb the vitamins and phytochemicals available in greens, and it's malnourishment that causes cravings for sweet foods. Greens are also full of fibre and help flush the system of toxins whilst making you feel full. They even increase the body's energy supply, which burns calories. So, if you're hungry between meals, you could always snack on veggies to up your intake.

Celery and cucumber sticks, as well as broccoli florets, make great snacks when combined with hummous, aioli or nut butters. Or you could juice a selection of green vegetables mixed with an apple or pear to provide a bit of sweetness. Or go all-out and have a green smoothie to boost your nutrient levels (see the recipe on page 222). However I take in my greens, I always choose organic.

Five-a-Day?

You should always consume as many portions of vegetables and fruits as possible too — up to seven or more! This can be made a bit easier if you make a green juice or make smoothies with fruits and green leaves to count as portions.

A recent study from the University of Warwick found that current UK government guidelines on the amount of fruit and vegetables we should be eating are woefully inadequate. Although for more than 20 years now the guidelines have suggested that we need to eat our five-a-day in order to stay healthy, seven to eight portions of 80g each is what we really should be aiming for, because it would be good for us both physically and mentally.

The Warwick study, which looked at the eating habits of 80,000 people in Britain, found a quarter eat just one or no portions of fruit and vegetables per day, while only a tenth consume seven or more.

However, the scientists also found that the people who eat between seven and eight portions of fruit and veg each day felt more cheerful, loved and optimistic about their futures. "This study complements... evidence of a long-known connection between, physical health and the consumption of fruit and vegetables.... Our findings are consistent with the need for high levels of fruit and vegetable consumption for mental health, not merely for physical health."[17]

Each government is responsible for setting health standards for its citizens. For instance, the Japanese, generally considered to be the healthiest nation on

Earth, are told to eat 13 portions of vegetables and four of fruit per day. The French guidelines are 10 portions a day, with the Canadians suggesting between five and 10. Meanwhile, the two countries with the most serious obesity problems — the US and UK — stick to advising its citizens five portions a day. Can you see the disconnect here?

Carbohydrates: Good or Bad?

The answer to this is both. Your body uses carbohydrates, or carbs for short, to make glucose — its primary energy source. Some carbs are good for the body, but then there are a lot of carbs that are bad.

As a rule, the more processed and refined the carbohydrate, the worse it is for you. Refined, or simple, carbohydrates include white flour, bread, pasta and potatoes, as well as sweets, sodas and desserts.

Complex carbohydrates, such as legumes, whole grains and sweet potatoes, contain longer chains of natural sugar molecules, so take longer to break down in the digestive system and help you to feel fuller for longer. And although the sugar content of fruit and vegetables classify them as simple carbohydrates, they also contain fibre, which changes the way the body processes their sugars and slows digestion as with complex carbs.

Although in recent years low-carb diets have been given much profile, they are a completely unsustainable way of maintaining permanent weight loss, even though massive losses in weight are achievable in the first few weeks of such programmes. For starters, this is because many low-carb diets also include elements of disease causing low-fat foods, such as margarine, other inflammatory vegetable oils and HFCS (glucose-fructose syrup), which as you now know makes you gain weight, especially visceral fat. So, although you may lose a lot of weight within the first few days or weeks on a low-carb diet, most of this will be from a loss of fluid in your cells. When muscle glycogen is depleted from lack of ingested carbohydrates, water is flushed from the body, which looks like rapid weight loss. As soon as you go back to your usual eating habits, all that water comes back — and then some.

Low-carb diets are also taxing to the body because they cause a big decrease in energy levels, allowing a way for fatigue to set in. They can also cause light-headedness and brain fog, which can make sticking to such diets unbearable for some, causing more stress and weight gain at the end of the ordeal. Remember, getting healthy *should not* be difficult, because your body's default mode is health.

In addition, a reduction in carbohydrate intake can impact your brain's serotonin levels (your 'feel good' hormone), which can put you at greater risk for mood imbalances and depression. So, if you choose not to eat carbs, no serotonin is made. Serotonin also has a part in helping you to feel satisfied (and not simply 'just full') after a meal.

Choose Wisely

For your optimum health, you should eat grains such as wholewheat flour and bread, brown rice, whole grain pasta, quinoa, whole oats, whole bulgur, amaranth and millet. Not only will these whole grains help to protect you against a range of chronic diseases, they are also nutritious, tasty and can be used in a variety of ways to keep your palate interested. Even 10 years ago, you would have been lucky to find brown rice at anything other than a non-traditional health food shop, but these days you can find quinoa in most supermarkets.

The easiest way to begin good carbohydrate eating habits is by starting the day with whole grains. If you're partial to a hot breakfast, why not try a warming bowl of porridge oats (not the instant kind) made with filtered water? Then add some fresh berries, a dollop of raw yogurt and a drizzle of maple syrup or raw honey for a satisfying and nourishing breakfast that will keep you full until lunch. If you're a cold cereal person, look for muesli with no-added-sugar that contains a wholegrain listed first in the ingredients.

Other good carb habits include using sweet potatoes instead of white potatoes when making mash or chips, or using brown rice, wholewheat bulgur (couscous), wheat berries, spelt, millet or barley in place of white rice at lunch or dinner.

Which Fat is Phat?

Fat is a far better source of energy for your body and brain than refined carbohydrates. In fact, fat is an extremely important part of your daily intake of nutrition, because two-thirds of your brain is made up of fat. Dietary fats are made up of fatty acids, some of which are used by the brain (after digestion in the small intestines) to synthesise brain and nerve tissue.

Cholesterol, a saturated fat much hyped as the cause of heart disease in the media, has an integral role in brain health. Therefore, a diet low in saturated fat has a role in impairing brain function.

In 1953, Dr Ancel Keys hypothesised (wrongly) that saturated fat and cholesterol caused heart disease. This is when hydrogenated vegetable oils and margarine (a coloured ingredient previously used in soap and candle-making) came into popular use, because they contained more mono- and poly-saturated fats, which were promoted by food manufacturers as good for heart health because they reduced blood cholesterol levels.

Blowing this common myth out of the water, Dr Mercola states:

> *"In a 1992 editorial published in the Archives of Internal Medicine, Dr. William Castelli, a former director of the Framingham Heart study, stated:*

'In Framingham, MA, the more saturated fat one ate, the more cholesterol one ate, the more calories one ate, the lower the person's serum cholesterol. The opposite of what... Keys et al would predict...We found that the people who ate the most cholesterol, ate the most saturated fat, ate the most calories, weighed the least and were the most physically active.'"[18]

Another 2010 study, published in the *American Journal of Clinical Nutrition*, found that a reduction in saturated fat intake must be evaluated in the context of replacement by other macronutrients, such as carbohydrates. The authors found that when saturated fat was replaced with a higher concentration of carbohydrates intake, especially refined carbs, then insulin resistance and obesity were exacerbated, along with heart disease.[19]

Therefore, eating fat and protein doesn't make you fat, carbohydrates do. This all means that the anti-saturated fat propaganda you previously knew as truth has been proven not to be. You know now that eating fat doesn't necessarily make you fat.

It's the *type* of fat that is the factor in making you fat.

In fact, it's absolutely imperative that you eat enough healthy fats in your diet to keep your hormones balanced and your blood sugar under control, which will help to prevent cravings.

The Good, Bad and Ugly

Good fats to begin adding into your new healthy eating lifestyle include extra virgin olive oil (never heat or it becomes toxic), virgin or raw coconut oil, raw grass-fed organic butter, grass-fed and wild meat/fish, raw (not roasted or salted) nuts, avocados, and sustainable palm oil. Another good habit is to completely avoid your use of vegetable oils and margarine-style spreads. Corn, cottonseed, soy, canola/rapeseed, safflower and sunflower oils can also be hydrogenated, the process of which turns them into trans fats.

You should be especially aware of rapeseed oil — in recent years, it has permeated the UK food scene and appears in most shop-bought and prepared foods.

Only virgin coconut oil should be used for cooking and baking, as it has a high smoke point. Do not use hydrogenated coconut oil for cooking, as the process used to hydrogenate the oil makes it turn to trans fat when you heat it.

Virgin or raw coconut oil also has antimicrobial properties, supports thyroid function, helps to strengthen your immune system, and helps build a strong metabolism, thus having the ability to be a fat that aids in weight loss. It's also a healthy saturated fat because it contains medium chain triglycerides (MCTs), which include a component called lauric acid, a powerful nutrient for your immune system. MCTs are readily used for energy by the body and are less likely to be stored as body fat compared with other fats.

Coconut milk is another good source of fat, while coconut flour can be used as a healthier flour option for baking, as it's extremely high in fibre and protein, and is also gluten-free.

Coconut oil can also be used on the skin or hair as a natural moisturiser without synthetic chemicals. You could even mix it with a few drops of essential oil when it has been gently warmed (coconut oil is solid below about

23°C). Virgin coconut oil is an all-round cupboard — and bathroom — essential fat you need to make friends with.

To round out your healthy fat intake, be sure to also include raw fats in your diet, such as avocados, extra virgin olive/hemp/flaxseed oils, raw dairy products and nuts (I do not include peanuts because a) they are actually legumes, and b) they are among the crops most heavily sprayed with pesticides). Avocados, which have been wrongly accused of causing fat, are high in monounsaturated fat, but they are also full of vitamins, minerals, micro-nutrients and antioxidants, which help your body maintain metabolic functioning for fat loss. This makes avocados are a fantastic energy source.

Healthy fats are also quite satiating, which means they keep you feeling fuller for longer. In addition, raw dairy, in the form of grass-fed butter, has high levels of a healthy fat called CLA, which has anti-cancer properties and has been shown to help burn abdominal fat. It also has an ideal balance of omega-3 and omega-6 fatty acids, which fight inflammation and can help balance hormones. Grass-fed butter also contains MCTs, helps satisfy your appetite and controls blood sugar levels.

Nutty News

You should also make friends with nuts, providing you don't have an allergy. Walnuts, almonds, pecans, pistachios, pinenuts, macadamia and Brazil nuts are generally between 75-90% fat in terms of a ratio of fat calories to total calories, but they're another type of healthy fat and also contain high levels of micronutrients such as vitamins, minerals and antioxidants. Nuts are also a good source of protein, which helps to control blood sugar and can aid in fat loss, and fibre.

Nuts can even help to maintain good levels of fat-burning hormones in your body (adequate healthy fat intake is vitally important to hormone balance), as well as help to control appetite and cravings so that you essentially eat fewer calories overall, even though you're consuming a high-fat food. My favourites are pecans, almonds, macadamias and walnuts, and by eating them in a variety of ways, you help to broaden the types of vitamins and minerals, and the balance of polyunsaturated to monounsaturated fats, you obtain.

Only buy raw nuts, as they will have more nutritional content of the healthy fats you need. You could always lightly toast them in a dry frying pan for a couple of minutes to enhance their flavour. Also, try to broaden your horizons beyond peanut butter (commercial brands have been found to contain pesticides and other chemicals such as flame retardant[20]) or make your own almond, cashew, pecan or macadamia butter to add variety to your diet (see recipe on page 231).

In addition to all these healthy fats, you should consider taking a good arctic Krill supplement. It is a clean source of animal-based omega-3, a deficiency of which is another contributory factor for chronic diseases.

Colon Cleanse

Now you know the types of food you'll need to be eating as part of your new healthy lifestyle, you will begin to introduce these foods into your life as part of the *Sizedrop 42 Days to a New You* plan. As you begin to do so, you will also begin to purge your body of the toxins it has accumulated through your consumption of processed food.

This will allow your body to benefit the most from the whole foods you'll now nourish it with.

The colon is usually considered the best place to start when removing toxins from the body, because that is where most accumulate. After that, other organs, such as the kidneys, liver and blood, can also be cleansed for better health and lasting weight loss. But your colon will be where the purging begins.

Depending on how severe your toxic buildup is, you may experience significant symptoms as the toxins are flushed out of your body in the first week of your new eating regime. You may get sick or experience flu-like symptoms, also know as a healing crisis. However, any discomfort you experience in the first few days will be worth it in the end. As your body begins to go into withdrawal from processed food, you might feel tired, your brain may feel foggy and you might be irritable.

During this time, it's important that you really pay attention to how your body feels. And after you finish the **_Sizedrop 42 Days to a New You_** plan, you should have a good think about how you will make eating in this way more sustainable to your individual needs. So, for example, it means you might have a glass of wine with your dinner or a black coffee in the morning. Just keep the junk out — for good. On the **Sizedrop 42 Days to a New You** plan, you will be detoxifying your body naturally and may find you begin to have more bowel movements than usual. This is all good. It means your colon is ridding itself of excess waste, which it definitely doesn't need.

Drinking fresh green juice may help to alleviate any detox symptoms. Besides being an easy way to consume more greens, juicing helps to accelerate the detoxification process. Remember: only use organic greens.

Drinking warm lemon water after waking up is a good habit you should start. Lemon juice, when mixed with lukewarm water, is a natural liver and kidney cleanser, both being major players in body detoxification. It also boosts your immune system and is alkalising to the body, which will help to break down fat deposits and toxins.

Another natural method for removing toxins from the body is sweating, which can happen through moderate exercise or by visiting a sauna. Used in conjunction with drinking lemon water and/or green juice, sweating is an easy way to help with detoxifying your body. And although it may be difficult for the first few days, detoxifying your body is something that you will definitely not regret.

Footnotes:

[16]Jeremy Laurance, "Death wish: Routine use of vital antibiotics on farms threatens human health", *The Independent*, 17 June 2011

[17]David G Blanchflower, Andrew J Oswald and Sarah Stewart-Brown, "Is Psychological Well-being Linked to the Consumption of Fruit and Vegetables?", University of Warwick and Dartmouth College, October 2012

[18]Dr Joseph Mercola, *The Forbidden Food You Should Never Stop Eating*, www.mercola.com, 1 September 2011

[19]Patty W Siri-Tarino et al, "Saturated Fatty Acids and Risk of Coronary Heart Disease: Modulation by Replacement Nutrients", *American Journal of Clinical Nutrition*, 14 August 2010

[20]Lynne Peeples, "Peanut Butter, Other Fatty Foods Found to Contain Fire Retardants in Recent Survey", *Huffington Post*, 31 May 2012

Chapter 6:
Exercise

Yes, it's necessary. Most people believe that weight loss is all about the calories: if you burn more calories than you take in, then you lose weight, and if you eat more calories than you burn, you'll gain fat. While this piece of logic may make sense, it is only partly true. What burns calories non-stop is actually the lean muscle mass that sits underneath your body fat. And it's this that allows you to take in more calories without weight gain.

However, the only effective strategy for sustainable weight loss includes exercise. Therefore, you're going to have to get used to the fact that you've got to start moving around more. Breaking into a sweat several times a week can help you to eliminate toxins via your skin, your largest organ. Your energy levels will also increase, because your body will be able to convert the whole food you'll be eating into energy faster with a regular dose of exercise.

In addition, exercise can help numb emotional and non-severe physical pain by releasing natural endorphins into the blood, which help to <u>alleviate</u> stress. Believe me, those endorphins came in very handy when I was recovering from the stress and grief at the loss of my Dad. Without the exercise, I don't know how I would have coped.

More than likely, it would have been with a prescription (or two) of antidepressants.

Because the fundamental issue of weight loss is still to burn more calories than you take in, you'll need to engage in some sort of activity that burns any excess. However, simple walking will do this, and by eating a wide and varied diet of fresh, organic whole foods, your body will be getting the nutrition it needs to function, so will be satisfied by what you eat.

Why You Need Muscle

It won't take long for your body to start adapting to the changes it will undergo. So, for instance, when you begin losing weight after the first three weeks on the *Sizedrop 42 Days to a New You* plan, if you don't begin adding some form of exercise into the mix, you'll increase the risk of losing lean muscle mass. This will have the effect of slowing down your metabolism and putting your body into fat-storing mode.

People who lose body fat as well as muscle mass, which happens to those who use a popular extreme high-protein and meal replacement weight-loss program, may at first experience drastic weight loss, but their facial features will also appear dry and gaunt, while their belly, arms and legs will usually be left with very saggy skin with no muscle tone. Worse yet, if these people overeat even a little bit, they will immediately start filling up on body fat once again.

Setting Goals

An important thing to remember when undergoing a weight loss program is that you need to incorporate the four elements involved — healthy food choices and a positive mindset, which we've covered, along with a supportive environment (which we'll get to soon) and physical activity.

As far as physical activity goes, setting realistic, specific and achievable goals for yourself can help in building the confidence you'll need to make the necessary leap to your desired weight. Write your realistic, specific and achievable goals down on a piece of paper and stick them up on the fridge so that you see it every day.

So, for example, if you decide you 'want to lose weight', unfortunately this means you probably won't achieve it. However, if you decide that you want to lose 14lbs and 2in around your waist in the next 12 weeks, then you will have specified an achievable goal to reach in a realistic time frame, which means you'll more than likely be motivated enough to continue working toward it.

I completely understand that the thought of exercise may seem daunting, or even scary, for some. I didn't partake in any form of exercise for almost 10 years, and when I started again, I only went to a yoga class once a week. These days, I still do a yoga class, but I've also added Pilates, weight training, whole body vibration training (PowerPlate), high-intensity cardio and a lot of walking into the mix. I now train 4-5 days a week, but even on those days when I rest, I make sure I get at least a 30-45-minute walk in somewhere.

Look at it this way: *how much do you actually value yourself?* I have a feeling there have been times when it's probably been not very much, which is why you're reading this. Therefore, you have to accept that this is simply another thing you will need to embrace in order to change your current situation.

If you currently do no exercise at all, your first step to achieving your new goal can be as small as taking some footsteps — for example, put this book down now and go for a 15-minute walk.

If you already do some exercise, then great! However, you should be aware that wearing yourself out with long periods of cardio, whether outside or at the gym, is boring for a reason — it does you no real good if you're looking to lose weight, and will only help if you are planning on running a marathon. Doing cardio exercises for long periods of time is also one of the worst ways to burn fat. How many times have I heard: "I've spent hours on the elliptical machine, riding a bike, using the rowing machine and I don't lose any weight"? Loads. And that's because it doesn't work if you're looking to burn fat.

If you're *really serious* about getting rid of fat, you'll need to introduce high-intensity interval training to your cardio routine, two to three times a week (see page 30).

Resistant to Resistance

Besides cardio, you're also going to need to introduce some resistance training to your activity routine. Yet the most common thing I hear from women when I mention this is: "But I don't want to have muscles like Arnold Schwarzenegger." Let's get this straight: unless you also decide to start taking steroids, which I *do not* advise, it is physically *impossible* for you to develop muscles like

Arnie simply by lifting weights. This is because women *do not* have the same levels of testosterone as men, and those high levels are needed to build huge, bulky muscle like that. Besides, resistance training is also an important factor in reducing your chances of developing osteoporosis, so you need to add it to your new exercise toolkit.

Breath Work

To top all this exercise stuff off, you'll get even further in helping to decrease your cortisol stress hormone levels by doing breathing and stretching exercises. Whenever you take part in any strenuous activity, you should *always* make sure that you also stretch properly afterward. Exercise is considered strenuous if it raises your heart rate and makes you sweat. Stretching afterward helps ensure you do your best to keep any injuries at bay.

Make sure you that you're breathing deeply whenever you are stretching to ensure increased blood flow to, and lactic acid removal from, the muscles. Besides helping to improve blood flow throughout the body, you can use deep breathing exercises to combat symptoms of anxiety and stress. Deep breathing is a common technique used to help people relax, reduce tension and relieve stress. When you engage in deep breathing activity, you also give yourself the ability to increase your mindfulness and awareness, which will help you to keep your mind and body functioning at their best.

Activity Ideas

The important thing to take away from all this is that whatever activity you do, it should be something you enjoy. That's because you'll be more than likely to stick to the activity, especially as you'll be feeling better and better by the day. Here are a few tips to get you started...

> **Pedometer:** Before you begin the ***Sizedrop 42 Days to a New You*** plan, I would like for you to buy a pedometer (you can find them for less than a fiver online at sites such as amazon.co.uk). Your *new cardio activity goal* is to take 10,000 steps a day — every day — for the next six months (and beyond). Yes — 10,000.
>
> On day one, you should wear your pedometer and go about your day as normal. If at the end of the day your step count is less than 5,000, then

you are considered to lead a *sedentary* lifestyle and are in serious need of taking control of your health. If the count is between 5,000 and 10,000, then you should increase your steps by 500 per day until you're reaching 10,000 on a daily basis. This means 70,000 steps a week are needed simply to maintain fitness.

HIIT: Or High-intensity interval training is the type of cardio training you need to be doing in order to torch the fat and promote the production of human growth hormone. You can use any cardio machine in the gym for this, although you can also use bodyweight exercises such as jumping jacks and mountain climbers, for example. HIIT should be done no more than three times a week to allow the muscles used to rest. Two popular HIIT protocols are Tabata and Dr Mercola's Peak 8 (see page 31).

Classes: Bodypump, Bodyattack, Bootcamps, Zumba, you name it... there are many group fitness classes run at gyms, outdoors and recreation centres all over the country. For example, if the free weights area in the gym has you fleeing in terror, why not try a Bodypump class to get your resistance training in? Or you like to dance? Then give Zumba or Bokwa a go?

Alternatively, most gyms have an induction system when you join so that you can be shown how to use the equipment and ask any questions you may have to one of the staff.

At home: Have access to a DVD player? There are loads of fitness DVDs on the market to buy or rent, so I'm sure you'll be able to find something that catches your fancy. If not, there's always YouTube and various fitness websites to search for ideas and exercise programs.

And you don't need to pump iron at a gym to carry out your resistance training. You can also make a circuit of simple exercises at home, such wall squats, plié squat jumps, lunges, pushups, triceps dips and planks.

And relax: Perhaps you might also want to consider finding a local yoga or Pilates class that you can attend (many yoga schools provide trial memberships for the first two weeks to a month), which will help with your stretching and breathing. Alternatively, you could download either a yoga, a Pilates or even a meditation app that will help guide you to breathe deeply before falling to sleep.

Feel Like S**t?

As a Thank You for reading this book, please visit www.feellikeshit.co.uk for your FREE BOOK BONUS

Chapter 7:
Accentuate the Positive

A positive thought:
I won't allow myself to think that my
physical appearance defines who I am as a person;
simply accept the fact that
I have worth as an individual.

Positive Attitude

Do you pick yourself apart or wish you looked a certain way? Do you compare yourself to airbrushed photos of your favourite celeb and feel that you always come up short? You need to begin letting go of these unrealistic notions and aim your focus on living an all-round healthier life. Losing weight obviously isn't easy or else everyone would be doing it, right? Sometimes even just thinking about it can seem too overwhelming.

But in order for the change you want to occur in the first place, you must be honest with yourself as to where you are now.

One key to successful permanent weight loss is to create a positive association with all of the hard work involved. So, for instance, with exercise it could be: "In an hour, at the end of my spin class, I'll feel so much better!" Or with healthy eating it could be: "If I choose to have the grilled chicken and asparagus for lunch, then I won't feel bloated all day." These will help you to stay on track when faced with temptations and hurdles. The fact is, having a negative attitude (even as innocuous as saying that you hate something) can actually make things harder for you — especially when it comes to seemingly impossible physical tasks and mental hurdles. So many of us are used to quitting before we have a chance to succeed — just so that we can have the excuse to say we never failed!

If you are not totally mentally prepared to increase your physical activity — as well as follow all the rules in *Sizedrop 42 Day to a New You* plan with a positive mind — then your chances for success are close to none.

You now know that it takes a lot more than just saying 'I want to lose a stone', 'I want to tone my thighs' or 'I want a tight bum' to get your mind ready for action to work its power on the body. Most people who are overweight because of the unhealthy food they eat *want* to 'be in shape' or 'be slimmer' than they are. But because they feel that they either won't or can't succeed, quite often they don't even try to make healthier food choices. They simply reach for what they're used to in the supermarket without thinking twice about it.

It's the same with exercise — we say we hate something, then refuse to do it, try it or 'stretch' ourselves. However, you should also keep in mind that hating something is the same as limiting yourself.

Emotional Crutches

Many people also put on weight because of negative emotional issues, such as depression, anxiety and anger. These are the major reasons why people indulge in too many sweets and refined carbohydrates, which, whether you're trying to lose inches or not, you now know are among the worst foods you can eat. They don't provide adequate enough nutrition and over-consumption will cause the body more harm than good.

To facilitate weight loss in a natural, healthy and permanent way, you must accept that where you have any physical imbalances (which manifest themselves through illness, disease, excess weight or a combination of all three), there has first been a non-physical causative factor. Basically this means there's a definite link between your emotions (whether positive or negative), your mental mindset (your habits) and your physical imbalances (illness, disease, excess weight). The great news is that it is possible to free your mind from the clutches of these negative emotions, so that you'll eventually feel more confident (more of this in Chapter 8). Changing your bad eating and activity habits to good ones will then become a breeze.

When I was overweight, I never really considered that I could ever be fit and healthy. Of course, it was something I dreamed of once in a while, but having been overweight since childhood, I never felt fitness was something I could realistically attain. I believed my GP when he said my physical decline over the years after glandular fever (skin rashes, oedema, frequent colds and flu, gluten intolerance, constipation and bloating, acid reflux, and so on) was due to the fact that I was getting older.

Of course, he would tell me to lose a few pounds, because of the diabetic theme that ran through the family, but never with any urgency. So I never did anything about it and accepted my decline as inevitable — like so many others do.

However, after the first two weeks of my detoxification process, I began waking up with a new lease of life. Increasingly, each day I would feel better than the last, which boosted my confidence enough so that when I first began working out at the gym, I started to feel better physically. And because I now felt better physically, mentally I started feeling better about myself too. And as I felt better mentally, I was able to put more effort into my workouts and start believing that I really *could* change my body.

Now, in the year I turn 49, my body is in better shape than it has ever been. And I still consider myself a 'work in progress'.

Trigger Points

Soon you too will begin replacing your bad food and activity habits with good ones. Seven days is all it takes to start a new beginning, free of negative emotional and mental triggers. The long-term rewards of physical and mental strength will provide you with what you deserve.

The challenge here is that you must become aware of any emotional and mental triggers that cause you to binge or make bad food choices in the first place. You must learn to monitor these triggers until your awareness reaches the point where you believe the action to shift them can actually happen. But also be aware that this is where most people give up — usually because they have a fear of the unknown, of what 'might' happen.

This is because in the beginning — when making the change in turning bad habits into good ones — it can be difficult to be detached and non-judgemental about our trigger issues. So, for instance, you may have had the best intentions of eating well today and getting to the gym after work, but if you found yourself running late this morning (and what was that excuse?), you didn't make your healthy lunch. Instead, you bought a sandwich from the kiosk at the station, which left you feeling bloated and depressed all afternoon. So you took a break at 4pm to buy chocolate, and because it was a bad day then bought a bottle of wine on the way home.

What happened to those good intentions? What trigger caused the negative behavioural pattern to re-emerge? When you learn to recognise the negative patterns, you'll learn to recognise the triggers.

And it's when we get past the trigger point that positive emotional and mental patterns can occur. While shifting your habits from bad to good during the *Sizedrop 42*

Days to a New You plan, you could try pretending that you are observing someone you don't know — just observe and don't judge. If it helps, you could it write down in a journal or a blog. For some people, this can provide the distance they need to be able to see themselves objectively. See what works for you.

Dear Diary

When I first began living a healthier lifestyle, I found it useful to keep a food diary. I was almost seven stone heavier than I am now, and it was only after I began writing down what I was eating could I see how terrible my mainly processed vegetarian diet really was (cheese, tofu, white pasta and bread, wine — and not many vegetables, ironically). I also realised I had ignored my poor eating because I was scared of changing my eating habits for the better. Even at the time, I knew it was a completely irrational way to think, because I didn't even know what I was scared of. I simply felt it wasn't possible to be anything other than 'big'.

With my food diary, I discovered that whenever I was bored, I used to snack, which led to my overeating. And I tended to snack when watching TV with a glass (or

144

three) of wine after dinner from the comfort of my sofa. So watching TV was another negative trigger issue that would make my brain shift my attention to junk food. These observations made me see the negative triggers that were causing me to abuse my own body.

I was able to stop the snacking by not buying unhealthy foods — if temptation wasn't in the cupboard, then it wouldn't cause a problem, would it? — and I find other things to do now besides mindlessly watching TV. By taking away the cause of my boredom and the temptation itself, I thereby eliminated the negative trigger issue.

And when you feel strong enough to have that kind of power over your cravings for negative nutrition, words can't describe the exhilaration you'll feel.

Once I began breaking the emotional way I felt about the negative foods and began accepting positive nutrition into my new lifestyle, it became obvious that there was nothing to be scared of and that I had everything to gain from being more healthy. I must admit this only came after much research on my part, as I felt the need to educate myself, and that left me feeling empowered enough to begin that first week of the rest of my life by leaving the self-abuse behind.

Focus Your Mind

Mental mindsets can also become trigger issues. For example, if you think negatively about your weight, this can actually cause you to eat more, which is the complete opposite of what you really want to do. Because there is such a strong connection between your thoughts, emotions and behaviours, low self-esteem and body image can also cause you to 'fall off the wagon' of your healthy eating regime. In order to truly *be* healthy, you have to *think* healthy.

Also know that this has nothing to do with perfection. More than likely in your quest for health, you'll reach a weight-loss plateau and won't be able to get the scale to budge. But instead of getting angry at what the scale is saying, why not take a minute to think about what the scale is not telling you — like what a strong and healthy individual you're becoming?

What you should be asking yourself is if you have more endurance than you did when you started? Have you lost inches from your waist? Do you feel better in your clothes? Don't be a slave to the scale. I ditched mine years ago. If you must, weigh yourself only once a week. The rest of the time just take note of the difference in how you're feeling.

Be aware that sometimes life has a way of throwing a curve ball. Also be aware that perfection never happens in real life. You will always do the best you can with this new information you have. And that's okay. You will always make progress toward your goals, however small, by improving your health and fitness.

Outside Influence

You may find that those closest to you may try to 'sabotage' your healthy efforts. For example, your hubby or partner may feel threatened by your new figure because you'll become more attractive to others. Or a good friend may feel jealous of your loss because she's not doing it herself. Or your mum may express her love through her calorie-laden Sunday roast, even knowing it may be harmful to your plans. If you feel you are being sabotaged, you need to find the inner strength to stick to your positive efforts.

You have to learn to be strong and say 'No' to food pushers. Simply reassure loved ones that you are the same person, just healthier. If they really do care about you, they will understand and be truly happy for you. Perhaps then you might even be able to encourage them to join you on the road to health.

You are in control. Of course, hiring a personal trainer or nutritionist, joining a local fitness group or eating healthy together with friends for encouragement can be used as aids to keep you motivated, as will initially trying to please a parent or spouse. However, these approaches will only motivate you at the beginning of your journey, so you can't rely on them for lifetime maintenance of a healthy weight. You need to learn to trust in yourself. You must also make sure you feed your brain with a healthy dose of positive thoughts daily.

Just as you'll be feeding your body with healthy food, the brain needs healthy, positive thoughts to thrive. So, for example, you could find a local yoga or meditation class to attend. Or perhaps you might download a meditation app onto your phone to help you keep your energy positive when you're out and about!

There's no doubt you will face mental challenges when you decide to change your lifestyle to a healthier one, so keeping your brain feeling healthy and positive is of the utmost importance. One way of achieving this is to visualise yourself as your healthiest you each day. This is because your journey to health will be more difficult if you can't see the end goal of how you want to both look and feel.

It's Up to You

Think about things this way: you didn't wake up one morning and all of a sudden find yourself overweight or obese. It simply didn't happen overnight. So, nor will the problem go away in a couple of weeks by popping a few 'slimming' pills or depriving yourself for 10 days with a severely restricting low-carb 'diet' that won't provide your body with all the nutrients it needs to function properly. Or by drinking energy protein shakes.

To truly overcome your health challenge, you have to be prepared to put the work in. How many inches or sizes you eventually lose will correspond to how much effort you put into making the right food choices and upping your activity levels. But it would be wise to take things in little steps so as not to make the challenge seem insurmountable. Introducing positive change and eliminating the negativity in your life will help you in these first steps to changing your life for a better, healthier one.

You have the power to make real changes to your health.

You simply have to believe it.

Positive Habit Forming in Five Easy Steps

1. Do Start: You've actually got to start a good habit or end a bad one. You can't reach day seven if you don't start at day one!

2. Stop the Excuses: Humans have become inherently lazy in today's gadget-run, car-dominated, processed food-consuming society. You'll likely be able to give yourself at least one reason not to start to change your bad habits to good ones. So, simply recognise your excuses for what they are — excuses — and instead find positive reasons to change them.

3. Write Them Down: And read them aloud to yourself every day to remind yourself of the reasons why you're doing them. Writing down your intentions will make them more tangible.

4. Keep Motivated: Dig out your old recipe books or search the internet for new ideas. Discuss and encourage your friends to join you for a local fitness group or class. Have a healthy lunch party with your girlfriends. Write a blog about your healthy journey. Use your imagination!

5. Announce Your Intentions: To everyone — even if they don't care. This isn't about them. It's about holding yourself accountable for your own actions. By telling everyone what you're doing, it will be harder for you to not do it!

Positive Habits to Start Today

✔ Write a food and exercise journal to keep motivated

✔ Blog about your weight loss efforts

✔ Aim to walk 10,000 steps per day

✔ Read something positive and life affirming

✔ Eat a vegetable or piece of fruit you've not tried before

✔ Meditate

✔ Go for a light jog outside in the fresh air

✔ Smile at people

✔ Laugh with a mate — or even on your own

✔ Work towards a goal

✔ Go to a yoga class

✔ Drink more filtered water

✔ Drink a green juice

✔ Take a bath

✔ Inhale essential oils

✔ Recite a mantra or positive affirmation

✔ Do something creative

✔ Don't consume aspartame, refined white sugar or MSG

✔ Eat breakfast

✔ Celebrate your successes

As a Thank You for reading this book, please visit www.feellikeshit.co.uk for your FREE BOOK BONUS

Negative Habits to Stop Today

✗ Smoking

✗ Swearing

✗ Eating non-organic meat

✗ Drinking too much alcohol

✗ Consuming non-organic dairy products

✗ Drinking soda

✗ Drinking coffee — especially decaffeinated

✗ Mindlessly watching TV

✗ Making excuses

✗ Being pessimistic/negative/gossiping about others

✗ Eating late/making bad food choices

✗ Binge eating

✗ Chewing gum

✗ Being late for meetings and appointments

✗ Eating non-organic chocolate

✗ Raising your voice

✗ Eating processed, fried and fast foods

✗ Taking drugs

✗ Causing or becoming involved in confrontation

✗ Using margarine

Chapter 8:
Tap for Weight Release

You should now have decided on the goals you want to set in order to bring healthy change into your life. Goal setting is just part of it, though. You need to *commit* to change. But to do this, you need to form new habits of your better choices, which I discussed in the previous chapter.

As a Thank You for reading this book, please visit www.feellikeshit.co.uk for your FREE BOOK BONUS

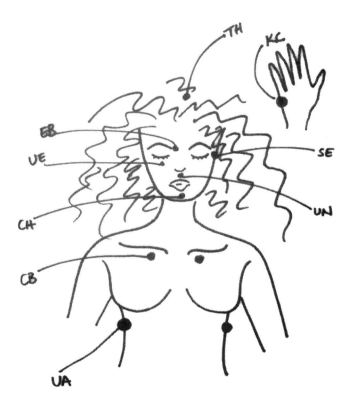

Diagram 1: Tapping points. Each point should be tapped on 5-10 times whilst reciting the corresponding pain or anxiety. When tapping on the points, use the index and middle fingers of each hand.

To make a new habit stick takes 21 days, because that's how long it takes to create the new neural path in your brain for the new action. This means that, unfortunately, you will mindfully have to make the right choice for three weeks, until your brain accepts the new habit.

This is also the reason most goals are never reached, because motivation from willpower alone generally fizzles out after a few days.

But don't despair, because it is entirely possible to make these changes without strong willpower. Instead of fighting urges and temptation, it is possible to make them go away. You can even make your mind believe that going to the gym and exercising is something you enjoy and desire, rather than dread.

Tap Away the Fat

Unfortunately, I didn't know about tapping (also known as EFT or Emotional Freedom Technique) when I started my weight loss journey, but I know it would have helped a great deal — even if only to deal with cravings on a bad day. I have, however, used tapping to great effect in recent months — to first admit to and then to control my deadly sugar addiction. It only takes a few minutes a day and is an amazing tool to add to your weight loss toolkit.

Tapping is a meridian-based energy therapy that helps to remove negative emotions that limit your potential. It was developed by Stanford University engineer and personal performance coach, Gary Craig, and is used as a tool to clear and resolve inner conflict in your brain. Specifically developed for use with those suffering from post-traumatic stress disorder, it combines Western psychology with the principles of Eastern acupuncture.

In regards to weight loss, you'll be able to use tapping to rid yourself of any stress you have about your current weight on a deep emotional and energetic level.

Each time you experience either emotional or physical trauma, it can potentially stay with you for the rest of your life, even if you think you've gotten over the incident. This is because chemicals are emitted by the brain's hypothalamus gland during a trauma and dock onto cell receptor sites, which inhibit proteins, vitamins and other nutrients from docking there. EFT helps to dislodge and clear these chemicals from the body, and

158

release your conscious mind of the associated negative thoughts. You will still recall an event as you did, but will no longer have negative feelings attached to it.

I know the idea of tapping may sound a bit new age and 'out there' to some people. However, all I ask is that you seriously consider adding it to the arsenal of weapons you're going to use kill your fat daemon once and for all.

Unlike affirmations, which will only work if you completely believe them, the best thing about tapping is that even if you don't quite believe in it, you will still be working on the meridian points stimulated to rid your body of any 'toxic' thoughts on a cellular level. So, even if your ego tells you there's no way that this is working, it still works.

I call that a win-win, don't you?

Tapping is a tool that can be used to deal with any sort of anxiety or fear you experience. The energy you create during a tapping routine 'allows' your body to release whatever negative, limiting or restrictive thoughts and beliefs you hold onto on a psychological level.

Take Sarah as an example: she 'thought' she wanted to lose weight, but after many attempts at dieting and exercising, she only seemed to put weight on. It was only when she decided to delve deeper, she realised that because she associated weight loss with losing something — her daily chocolate fix — she generally felt down every time she went on a diet, which was never going to work. When Sarah learned about tapping and how it could help her to release her restrictive beliefs around her weight issues, the weight began coming off.

If you release something, there is no restriction given to it. So, if you learn to 'release' the fat you don't want by tapping, you can begin to 'allow' the extra weight to leave your body. You've got to admit that this is a very powerful tool to use with your new nutritional and activity regime. You should aim to do a round of tapping at least once a day or whenever any negative thoughts begin pestering your mind. Like brushing your teeth, the more you tap the negativity away, the sooner you will achieve peace regarding whatever it is you're tapping about. For more information on tapping, there are many resources available on the internet. Below is a tapping sequence you can use to get started,

Tapping Sequence

Get and piece of paper and pen ready, then go to sit up straight in a comfortable chair, with both feet on the ground and take a deep breath in. Decide on the anxiety or belief you want to tap away – for example, 'sometimes it feels like I'll never lose weight'). Then, on a scale of 1 to 10, with '1' being 'I'm feeling calm' and '10' being 'OMG I just might be sick I'm so stressed', write down on the piece of paper the number that you feel. If it's a '6' or above, then it's time to get tapping!

Begin with the Karate Chop (KC) point (it doesn't matter which hand you use). The KC point is used as your 'set up' statement and you can tap it with the pads of the fingers of the opposite hand.

The other points in the sequence (see diagram on page 156) include the Top of Head (TH), Eyebrow (EB), Side of Eye (SE), Under Eye (UE), Under Nose (UN), Chin Point (CH), Collarbone (CB) and Under Arm (UA).

Tap these points with the index and middle fingers of both hands. During the sequence, you tap each energy point between five and 10 times.

Feel Like S**t?

At the end of the tapping routine, take another deep breath in and check in with how you feel. Has the bad feeling lessened any? If it has, then great! Or does it still stir up ill feeling? On the scale of 1 to 10, if it's more than a '4', then you should do another round of tapping until the negative feelings decrease.

KC Even though I don't like what I see in the mirror, I completely accept and love myself (even if you don't believe it yet!)

EB I don't feel good in my clothes

SE My thighs rub and that sometime causes me pain

UE I feel bloated and ugly most of the time

UN I don't want to do change my eating habits

CH But I am going to do it

CB It might not even work

UA And even if I lose this weight

TH It'll probably all just come back on again

EB That's what happened the last time

SE And all the times before that

UE And what about all that ugly, loose skin?

UN Isn't it worse to have that than just to stay fat?

CH Besides, everyone knows that *real* women are

162

voluptuous and sexy

CB And no-one wants to cuddle a bag of bones

UA Which is what would happen if I release the weight

TH I love my curves, because they make me voluptuous

EB But maybe I can just learn to be patient with my body as it transforms

SE Maybe I can choose to eat whole foods instead of taking the easy option and getting a takeaway

UE Maybe I can also find an activity that I enjoy to help with the release

UN And I can walk some more every day, because I can always find 10 minutes for myself

CH I think I *can* do this for my body

CB I think I *need* to do this for my body

UA I choose to be healthy for myself, so that I can do the things that I want to do in this life

TH It feels good to be aware of what I eat, so that I get all the nutrition I need for my cells to thrive

Feel Like S**t?

Chapter 9:
Time to Take Action

You're now armed with all the information you need to start getting healthy, releasing the excess flab you're carrying around and feeling better about yourself in general. You've been told the truth about how Big Food is not in the business of keeping you healthy; it's in the business of making profits for its shareholders. You now know the truth about how the processed 'diet' meal replacement products of Big Weight Loss don't work; their low-fat/low-carb/high-protein diet bars/packet soups/shakes might see you lose weight at first, but your body will soon react to the calorie restrictions and you'll probably gain it all back... and then some.

I've explained to you the truth about how hours of cardio exercise can keep you flabby and that it's better to do a mix of short, intense intervals, along with some resistance training, breathing and stretching. And you know that starving yourself doesn't work, because you'll always gain back whatever water you initially lost, along with some brand new fat cells. You should also now believe it's not an impossibility that you yourself can live a life of health, because by following the *Sizedrop 42 Days to a New You* plan, you will experience:

- ✓ An increase in energy levels
- ✓ A boost to your immune system
- ✓ Clearer skin and nails, along with thicker hair
- ✓ Better sleep quality
- ✓ A renewed vitality for life
- ✓ An increase in self-confidence and self-love

Remember that every day is another step achieved, and you should be proud of yourself for even getting this far. It means you've already made some of the mindset changes needed to do this. But I must be honest with you — there will be times when you will fall off the wagon of wellness. Life can have a way of throwing up stressful situations you must deal with, usually when you least expect it. And whatever stress it is might just have you reaching for whatever comfort food, drink or stimulant you would have turned to in the past. You might even binge.

That is where you have to end it, though!

If you want to live with optimum health, then you're going to have sacrifice the instant gratification of eating (and overeating) junk, taking stimulants (coffee, caffeine, cigarettes, pharmaceutical and recreational drugs) and not moving much.

Ups and Downs

I'm only human, and I've had my ups and downs since becoming stronger and healthy. Within the first 18 months of my career as a fitness professional, I burned myself out and started picking up injuries, so I couldn't train myself optimally. This lead to feeling down and reaching for organic gingerbread cake (I told myself that because it was made with organic molasses, it was ok. I now know that if you are insulin sensitive or have any sort of blood sugar disorder, no matter whatever form it's in, sugar is sugar. And it will make you sick with inflammation, metabolic syndrome, diabetes and cancer.).

I gained back 12lbs when I reached my lowest ebb — about four months in. Besides the extra belly fat, I also suffered weeks of sleepless nights due to night sweats. Throughout the ordeal, though, in the back of my mind I knew I had the ability to turn things around because of how far I had come, and so I had to get back on it. Again, I had to snap myself out of my self-pity and take control of the sugar addiction. And it has to be said, that 12lbs was almost harder to lose than the previous 6st.

It's all about the choices you make. What I'm saying is that even on the days you make the conscious decision to have that scrumptious piece of cake, you've got to get back on your health trip at your next meal. You musn't allow a bad food day to turn into a bad food week — or month, or year.

Change can be painful and often involves some struggling. But each time you push yourself beyond your comfort zone, you'll grow even more confident in your abilities. You cannot paint a masterpiece if you don't pick up a paintbrush. Keep a food diary for the next few weeks until you are comfortable and confident in what you're doing. Logging your food and drink intake will constantly confirm everything you are doing right, or highlight where you may need to do some more work.

Listen to Your Body

Ditch the scales and use how you feel, and how your clothes are fitting, as guides on how you're getting on. You are worth being healthy, confident, loved and strong. So keep moving and working towards your goals.

Stop listening to the little voices in your head that tell you not to take action. That will be your self-sabotage working. Don't listen to what others have to say about what you're doing either. They may have a vested interest in sabotaging your efforts, even if it's unconscious (be aware that many people don't like seeing others lose weight successfully, because it puts their lack of 'willpower' on show).

Taking action means you don't *talk* yourself into doing it — you just *do* it. Taking action means you don't *make excuses* as to why you should do it later — you just *do* it. You have to take action over and over and over again until it becomes automatic. This is when it will become a way of life, an unconscious habit.

When you first begin to take action, it will probably feel uncomfortable. You may even feel as if you've failed at the first hurdle. That's fine, you simply need to take more time to allow your new habits to ingrain themselves into your being. This simply takes practise. Do a tapping sequence to clear any procrastination or self-sabotage. Do small good things every day and they will eventually become good habits. Simple.

Learn from any mistakes you make (we're all human, so it will happen); simply try to do things differently if something doesn't work for you, or even try something else. You have to practise the habit of taking action. You

170

have to do it over and over and over again until it starts feeling natural and comfortable.

You're Your Own Hero

Be an action hero. At some point or other, we've all thought about giving up on something. No matter what the task, you will have reached a point where you could no longer see the light at the end of the tunnel. But now you've got to have a word with yourself, because only you can do this.

Instead of thinking about giving up, just do something, however small, that takes you towards your goal. So, for example, you can use the stairs at work rather than the lift. Or get off the bus a couple of stops early. Or save the money from your daily coffee to buy something special to celebrate Do something that perhaps takes you out of your comfort zone a little; it will be all the better for you in the end if it does.

After completing the *Sizedrop 42 Days to a New You* plan, you'll probably wonder what all the fear was about, because it actually feels good to be able to do something that takes you anywhere you haven't been before, or in a long while. And, as with anything, over time you'll find that it gets easier while your daily little successes happen (I didn't eat any sugar today!).

Take things one step at a time, setting small goals and using your tools to get there. I *know* you can do it!

Your Daily Action List

Visualisation: If you cannot visualise yourself in perfect health, then you are seriously undermining your weight loss efforts. You should spend at least three to five minutes each day visualising yourself in a favourite outfit, or doing something new or fun you'll be able to do with your new body. You can even do this while you're exercising.

Don't stress about it, though. Just find the image of the ideal you, and let it go after a few minutes. Close your eyes and just imagine yourself in great shape doing something you love. Unifying the mind and body will drastically increase your chances of reaching your healthy target.

Drink Water: Drink 2-3 litres of filtered water each day, adding 500ml for each 30 minutes of strenuous exercise you may do (if it makes you sweat). According to Ayurvedic principles, sipping on hot water helps to cleanse the lymphatic system and combat cravings, which can aid in fat loss.

A good daily habit to get into is to have a cup of hot water and fresh squeezed lemon upon rising. Although lemons themselves are acidic, this drink helps the body become more alkaline, which in turn helps to maintain pH balance and promotes optimum health.

Evening Meal: Don't eat your evening meal any later than 8pm. This is because eating too close to bedtime disrupts your body's natural cycle. Food also takes time to digest, so allow your body to do this during the day so that it can rest properly at night. If you go to bed early, say before 10pm, then you should have your final meal no later than 7pm.

Chew Your Food Well: This will happen naturally, because it is impossible to eat whole foods without chewing properly. You will also become more conscious about what you put into your mouth. Chewing thoroughly aids in the digestion process, which in turn makes you feel fuller faster.

Saying Is Believing: Begin reciting your affirmations aloud in front of a mirror (I love my strong, healthy and sexy body; I love myself; I only eat nutritious food to give my body the nutrients it needs to function properly; and so on). Talking to your brain is a powerful tool. The more you say something and truly believe it, then the more real it will become.

Set A Budget: You have to accept that you may have to spend more for good-quality meat, fish, fruit and vegetables. However, your investment in yourself to get healthy, as well as achieve weight loss and renewed health, will pay for itself in years to come. Your new lifestyle will automatically see you cutting back on expenses in other areas, such as morning coffees, cigarettes, alcohol, the latest weight-loss fad and clothing you don't need. When you make smart choices and invest in your future, you can become your best self easily.

Write It Down: Write down your weight loss goals, both big and small. Write down your health-related goals. Do you want to fit back into your skinny jeans in the back of the cupboard? Write it down. Want to knock them dead at your school reunion? Write it down.

Support Network: Read other books about healthy living — for suggestions, see page 239. There are many books available on weight loss and health, in general. Reading something that is positive forms a great impression on your being. You'll soon begin to absorb the information and align your healthy intentions accordingly. You could also join an online forum or community and get support for your new lifestyle that way. You can even ask questions.

Or perhaps you start attending a local meet-up group that focuses on nutrition and health, so that you can meet others who are doing what you do. Don't worry about being judged or criticised. Remember to step outside your comfort zone! When you totally immerse yourself in changing your lifestyle, the weight will fall off without you really even noticing.

Accountability: Now that you've decided that health is your new journey, start sharing what you are doing with others. When you begin to vocalise your goals to others, not only do they become more real to you, but you'll now also be held accountable for what you have shared.

Begin by sharing with those closest to you, as you never know, you might also find a buddy to share the journey with. Do, however, be aware that not everyone will be on the same page as you. In fact, some people (including those closest to you) may be downright hostile about what you're doing.

This has nothing to do with them, though. This is your health journey, and if they're not onboard, then so be it. Tell them 'Thanks for sharing' and move on with your daily healthy intentions, step by step — until they become your new habits.

Personal Best

All you need to do now is make a commitment to yourself during these next 42 days in your life. You must follow the rules religiously, if you want to change the way you look enough. It really shouldn't feel like a chore, but the start of a new journey.

Your only alternative is an inactive life of prescription medication, Type 2 diabetes, high blood pressure, coronary heart disease and cancer.

How much is your life worth, anyway? Make the change now and don't give up. It's just 42 days out of your life.

Go on... I dare you not to feel better by the end of it — that's when you'll realise this is just the beginning of the rest of your life.

So, right this minute, you're going to commit to doing one thing to take you to your ultimate health goal. Just one. Make it small to start. For instance, you could go through your cupboards and throw out anything that contains HFCS or aspartame — such as diet soda, flavoured crisps, flavoured water, sugar-free products, yogurt, ketchup, cereals and chewing gum. Or find out when and where your local farmers' market is and schedule the next one into your diary. Or get a friend to join you on your walk to help you reach your 10,000-step target. You get the picture. It's time to stop procrastinating and take action.

Just do it...

If I can, then I sure as shit *know* you can too!

Chapter 10:
Sizedrop Natural Weight Loss Solution's
42 Days to a New You Food Plan

Laid out on the following pages is my *Sizedrop 42 Days to a New You* plan. Through lots of education, research, <u>trial</u> and error, I managed to completely turn my life around from one of chronic illness, depression, stress and obesity to one of health and a lightness of being that I had never before imagined. This is the fruit of my experience.

I recommend that you take a couple of days to read through it and work out how you're going to handle the changes it will bring, go shopping to buy the foods that you'll need, then commit yourself 100% to getting through these six weeks. Have a look around at other places to buy your food rather than supermarkets. For instance, perhaps there's an ethnic supermarket nearby, which is a good place to find exotic vegetables (and although they may not be organic, they likely won't be GMO either).

Filling out your food diary is a great way of keeping an eye on what you're eating — especially the effects that different amounts of carbohydrates, fats and proteins have on the way you feel.

Remember that you are the only person who can be held responsible for your health. Listen to what your body (not your brain — or anyone else) is trying to tell you about the choices you will make.

Once you understand that, the world will gradually become a different place — in a much better way — and you'll be in the driver's seat, taking control of your own health, not just for 42 days, but for the rest of your life!

Get the Balance Right

Each plate of food you eat should consist of about 40% high-quality protein, 40% complex carbohydrate (including as much green vegetables as possible) and 20% fat. A good measure for quantities is your own hand, because it is relative to your stomach size, so makes a great measuring device of how much food you should ingest. Your protein shouldn't be any larger than your palm. You should include a fist-sized portion of vegetables. If extra carbs are included, they should only fill a cupped hand size and should not be refined (white). Your fat quantity should be the size of your thumb.

Days 1-7: The first week of the *Sizedrop 42 Days to a New You* plan will make you aware of exactly what it is you are eating. From days 1-7, you should record everything you eat for breakfast, lunch and dinner, as well as any snacking between meals in the Food Diary on page 185.

You should also record any beverages you drink, including water, tea, coffee and alcohol. And if your morning coffee includes added syrups, sugar, cream and so on, then this should also be recorded.

Days 8-27: The next 20 days will be the hardest on the *Sizedrop 42 Days to a New You* plan. This is the detoxifying stage, also known as a healing crisis, and you may find that you experience muscle aches, mucous discharge, headaches, coated tongue, nausea, weakness, cravings, constipation, diarrhoea, gas, irritability, disrupted sleep and flu-like symptoms. However, this is a completely normal process to go through as the body releases toxins from the fat cells to be flushed out by the colon, kidneys and liver.

To cope with a healing crisis, make sure you drink plenty of fresh water, homemade green juices (see page 220 for recipe suggestions) and herbal teas to help flush out toxins. Hot water and fresh lemon is also a great detoxifier. And use a sauna if you can, as sweating is an easy way to release toxins from the skin. If you are feeling lethargic or tired, your body is telling you that you need to rest, so do so. Any healing crisis shouldn't last for more than a few days. To make sure the detox process works and to give your body the best chance of healing, follow the **No-Go, Foods to Avoid** and the **All You Can Eat** food lists to the letter. If you are ever hungry, simply have a snack from the **All You Can Eat** list. You should not experience hunger on the *Sizedrop 42 Days to a New You* plan.

Days 28-42: In the final 15 days on the *Sizedrop 42 Days to a New You* plan, you begin to introduce a few more foods into the repertoire. By now you should already be feeling a renewed sense of energy, clearer skin and a relief from gas and/or bloating, as well as any previous symptoms of food intolerance and allergies. Again, please follow the **No-Go, Foods to Avoid** and **All You Can Eat** food lists to the letter.

All that's left now is for you to get started.

Feel Like S**t?

The legal disclaimer bit:

It is not claimed that the **Sizedrop 42 Days to a New You** plan will treat, or is intended to treat, any medical condition. The **Sizedrop 42 Days to a New You** plan is undertaken entirely of your own choice, at your own risk, in the full understanding that the dietary advice given is in no way designed individually for you. If you believe that by following the **Sizedrop 42 Days to a New You** plan you experience adverse side effects, or that it is harmful to you in any way whatsoever, then stop immediately and seek medical advice.

The author does not assume any responsibility or liability for any adverse effects or consequences you experience either directly or indirectly as a result of following (or not) the advice or suggestions made in the **Sizedrop 42 Days to a New You** plan.

Sizedrop 42 Days to a New You Food Diary

	Breakfast	Lunch	Dinner	Snacks and Beverages
Day 1				
Day 2				
Day 3				
Day 4				
Day 5				
Day 6				
Day 7				

Sizedrop 42 Days to a New You Food Diary

	Breakfast	Lunch	Dinner	Snacks and Beverages
Day 8				
Day 9				
Day 10				
Day 11				
Day 12				
Day 13				
Day 14				

Sizedrop 42 Days to a New You Food Diary

	Breakfast	Lunch	Dinner	Snacks and Beverages
Day 15				
Day 16				
Day 17				
Day 18				
Day 19				
Day 20				
Day 21				

Sizedrop 42 Days to a New You Food Diary

	Breakfast	Lunch	Dinner	Snacks and Beverages
Day 22				
Day 23				
Day 24				
Day 25				
Day 26				
Day 27				
Day 28				

As a Thank You for reading this book, please visit www.feellikeshit.co.uk for your FREE BOOK BONUS

Sizedrop 42 Days to a New You Food Diary

	Breakfast	Lunch	Dinner	Snacks and Beverages
Day 29				
Day 30				
Day 31				
Day 32				
Day 33				
Day 34				
Day 35				

As a Thank You for reading this book, please visit www.feellikeshit.co.uk for your FREE BOOK BONUS

Sizedrop 42 Days to a New You Food Diary

	Breakfast	Lunch	Dinner	Snacks and Beverages
Day 36				
Day 37				
Day 38				
Day 39				
Day 40				
Day 41				
Day 42				

Sizedrop 42 Days to a New You Step Counter

	Sun	Mon	Tues	Wed	Thurs	Fri	Sat
Week 1							
Week 2							
Week 3							
Week 4							
Week 5							
Week 6							

Your aim is to take *at least* 10,000 steps per day. If on your first day you take less than 4,000 to 5,000 steps, you should aim to increase your steps by 500 each day until you can easily do around 10,000 on a regular or daily basis.

Sizedrop 42 Days to a New You Food Plan: Days 8-27

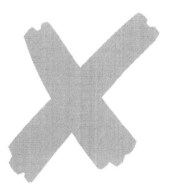

No-Go

The following foods **are not allowed** on days 8 to 27. If a food is not on either of the other two lists (for days 8 to 27) or is on this one, then put it out of temptation's way, or better yet, throw it in the bin!

Meat and Poultry

Bacon
Burgers
Ham
Heart
Hotdogs
Kidney
Liver
Offal
Pork
Processed meats
Sausages

Fish and Seafood

Caviar
Clams
Cod
Crab
Crayfish
Eel
Haddock
Halibut
Lobster
Mussels
Octopus
Oysters
Plaice
Prawns
Salmon (farmed)
Swordfish
Trout (farmed)
Tuna

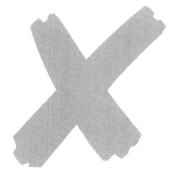

Nuts and Seeds

Peanuts

193

Grains

Amaranth
Barley
Buckwheat
Kamut
Millet
Oat
Quinoa
Oat
Rice
Rye
Spelt
Wheat

Fruit

Apricot
Cherries
Currants
Dates
Figs
Grapes
Kiwi
Mango
Melon
Nectarine
Orange
Papaya
Peaches
Pear
Pineapple
Plums
Pomegranate
Prunes
Raisins
Rhubarb
Strawberries

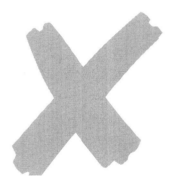

As a Thank You for reading this book, please visit www.feellikeshit.co.uk for your FREE BOOK BONUS

Vegetables and Legumes

Aduki beans
Black beans
Broad beans
Butter beans
Chickpeas
Green peas
Haricot beans
Kidney beans
Lentils
Mung beans
Mushrooms
Potatoes (white)
Soybeans (edamame)
Sweetcorn
Tofu

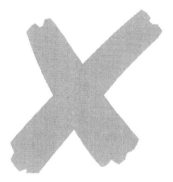

Dairy

Cow's milk yogurt
Cow whey
Pasteurised cow's milk
Brie
Camembert
Cheddar cheese
Cottage cheese
Cream (single/double/whipped)
Cream cheese
Edam cheese
Gouda cheese
Gruyere cheese
Ice cream
Mozzarella cheese
Parmesan cheese
Ricotta cheese
Sour cream
Swiss cheese

As a Thank You for reading this book, please visit www.feellikeshit.co.uk for your FREE BOOK BONUS

Oils and Fats

Margarine
Rapeseed/Canola oil
Safflower oil
Salted butter
Sunflower oil
Vegetable oil

Herbs, Spices and Seasonings

Chocolate/Cocoa
Ketchup
Mayonnaise
Salt (table/iodised/low sodium)
Soy sauce
Sugar
Sweetener (aspartame/saccharin)
Vanilla extract
Vinegar (malt)

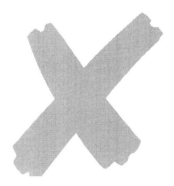

Beverages

Beer
Coffee
Fruit juice
Oat milk
Rice milk
Soft drinks (carbonated)
Soy milk
Sparkling water
Tea (black)
Tap water
Wine (red/white/rosé/sparkling)
Spirits (alcohol)

Sizedrop 42 Days to a New You Food Plan: Days 8-27

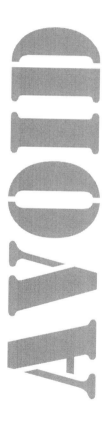

Avoid

The following foods are only to be **eaten in moderation** on days 8 to 27. For instance, the meat and fish listed below should be eaten no more than once every 3-4 days. In all other cases, you should eat smaller amounts than usual if using most days — for example, when using bananas for smoothies or sheep cheese for salads.

Always buy organic whenever possible.

Meat and Poultry
Beef
Buffalo
Lamb

Fish and Seafood
Anchovy
Mackerel
Sea bass
Squid

Fruit
Banana

Vegetables
Plantain

Dairy
Feta cheese
Goat's milk yogurt
Goat's cheese
Halloumi cheese
Roquefort cheese
Sheep's cheese
Sheep's yogurt

Herbs, Spices and Seasonings
Raw honey

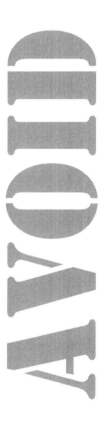

Sizedrop 42 Days to a New You Food Plan: Days 8-27

All You Can Eat

On days 8 to 27, you are **allowed to eat all** of the following foods listed below. There's **no counting calories**, so simply choose from the list to satiate your appetite.

As always, buy organic whenever possible.

Meat and Poultry

Chicken
Duck
Goat
Goose
Pheasant
Quail
Rabbit
Turkey
Venison

Fish and Seafood

Herring/Kipper
Wild Salmon
Sardine
Snapper
Wild Trout

Nuts and Seeds

Almonds
Brazil nuts
Cashew nuts
Chestnuts
Hazelnuts
Macadamia nuts
Pecans
Pinenuts

Fruit

Apples
Blackberries
Blueberries
Coconut
Cranberries
Grapefruit
Lemon/Lime
Raspberries
Watermelon

Vegetables and Legumes

Artichokes (globe and Jerusalem)
Asparagus
Aubergine
Avocado
Beetroot
Bok choy
Broccoli
Brussel sprouts
Butternut squash
Cabbage
Capers
Carrots
Cauliflower
Celeriac
Celery
Chard
Courgette
Cucumber
Fennel
Garlic
Ginger
Green beans
Kale
Leeks
Lettuce (iceberg/romaine)
Mangetout
Onions
Parsnips
Peppers
Pumpkin
Radish
Rocket
Spinach
Spring greens
Sprouts (aduki, alfalfa, lentil)
Sweet potato
Tomatoes
Watercress

Dairy
Eggs
Goat whey

Oils and Fats
Butter (unsalted)
Coconut butter/oil
Flax or Hemp seed oil
Palm oil (sustainable)
Sesame oil
Extra virgin olive oil
Ghee

Herbs, Spices and Seasonings
Basil
Bay
Cardamon
Carob
Cayenne
Chilli
Chives
Cloves
Coriander
Cumin
Curry powder
Fennel
Horseradish
Lemongrass
Mint
Mustard
Oregano
Paprika
Rosemary
Turmeric
Sea salt
Vinegar (apple cider/balsamic)

Beverages

Almond milk
Coconut milk
Coconut water
Herbal teas
Vegetable juices (unpasteurised)
Water (filtered or bottled)

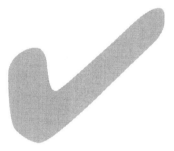

Days 8-27

Menu suggestions

Breakfast
Poached egg with spinach and grilled tomatoes
Mushroom and herb omelette
Goat's milk yogurt and berries
(optional: add coconut chips or mixed seeds)
Apple, banana and berry smoothie
Kippers with grilled tomatoes

Lunch
Grilled herring fillets with sweet potato mash
Leek frittata with tomato and basil salad
Carrot and cumin soup
Roasted butternut squash with spinach and goats cheese
Grilled sardines with steamed broccoli

Dinner
Roast lemon chicken breast, baked root vegetables and green beans
Pan-fried steak, sweet potato wedges (recipe on page 223) and green beans
Chilli beef, cabbage and pepper stir-fry
Grilled lamb chops with cherry tomatoes and stir-fried vegetables
Grilled halloumi cheese with sweet potato wedges (recipe on page 223) and salad

Snacks
Apple and almond butter (recipe on page 231)
Avocado, roasted mixed seeds and vinaigrette
Green vegetable juice (recipe on page 220)
Aubergine babaganoush with crudites

Note: these suggestions are just that — suggestions. They show you how you can eat, not how you must *eat.*

Need to know

During the first few days of the *Sizedrop 42 Days to a New You* plan, you may experience withdrawal symptoms — such as a headache due to no caffeine or sugar. These are symptoms of detoxification and are completely normal. Just make sure that you drink plenty of filtered (or bottled) still water throughout the day to help flush out any toxins from your body. Aim to drink at least 2-3 litres a day.

You should begin your day with a large glass of water with a squeeze of lemon to help support the liver during this process.

You should also aim to eat every three to four hours in order to boost your metabolism. And you should learn to only eat until you feel comfortably satisfied (that's about 85% full) — not until your sides are bursting!

REMEMBER: if a food is not allowed on days 8-27, then don't consume it!

Sizedrop 42 Days to a New You Food Plan: Days 28-42

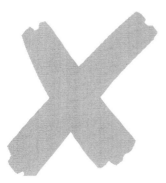

No-Go

The following foods **are not allowed** on days 28 to 42. If a food is not on either of the other two lists (for days 28 to 42) or is on this one, then put it out of temptation's way, or better yet, throw it in the bin!

Meat and Poultry
Bacon
Burgers
Ham
Heart
Hotdogs
Kidney
Liver
Offal
Pork
Processed meats
Sausages

Fish and Seafood
Caviar
Clams
Eel
Mussels
Oysters
Prawns
Salmon (farmed)
Swordfish
Trout (farmed)
Tuna

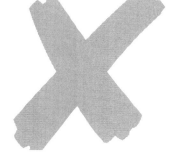

Nuts and Seeds
Peanuts

Grains
Oat
Rice (white)
Wheat

Fruit
Currants
Dates
Figs
Prunes
Raisins

Vegetables and Legumes
Mushrooms
Potatoes (white)
Soybeans (edamame)
Tofu

Dairy
Pasteurised cow's milk
Ice cream

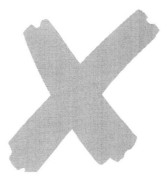

Oils and Fats
Butter (salted)
Corn oil
Margarine
Rapeseed oil (canola)
Safflower/Sunflower oil
Soybean oil
Vegetable oil

Herbs, Spices and Seasonings
Chocolate/Cocoa
Ketchup
Mayonnaise
Salt (table/iodised/low sodium)
Soy sauce
Sugar
Sweetener (aspartame/saccharin)
Vanilla extract
Vinegar (malt)

As a Thank You for reading this book, please visit www.feellikeshit.co.uk for your FREE BOOK BONUS

Beverages

Beer
Coffee
Fruit juice
Oat milk
Rice milk
Soft drinks (carbonated)
Soy milk
Sparkling water
Tea (black)
Spirits (alcohol)

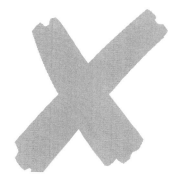

Sizedrop 42 Days to a New You Food Plan: Days 28-42

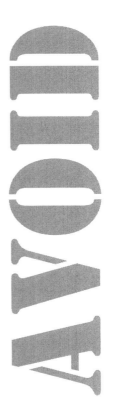

Avoid

The following foods are only to be **eaten in moderation** on days 28 to 42. For instance, the meat and fish listed below should be eaten no more than once every 3-4 days. In all other cases, you should eat smaller amounts than usual if using most days — for example, when using bananas for smoothies or goat's cheese for salads.

Always buy organic whenever possible.

Meat and Poultry
Beef
Buffalo
Lamb

Fish and Seafood
Anchovy
Cod
Crab
Crayfish
Halibut
Haddock
Mackerel
Octopus
Plaice
Sea bass
Squid

Grains
Barley
Buckwheat
Millet
Quinoa
Rice (brown and wild)
Rye
Spelt

Fruit
Banana
Guava
Mango
Melon
Nectarine
Oranges
Peaches
Rhubarb
Strawberries

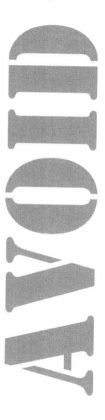

Vegetables
Mushrooms
Plantain
Sweetcorn

Dairy
Brie
Camembert
Cheddar cheese
Cottage cheese
Cream
Cream cheese
Cow's milk yogurt
Edam
Feta cheese
Goat's milk yogurt
Goat's cheese
Gouda
Halloumi cheese
Mozzarella
Parmesan cheese
Ricotta cheese
Roquefort cheese
Sheep's cheese
Sheep's milk yogurt
Sour cream
Swiss cheese

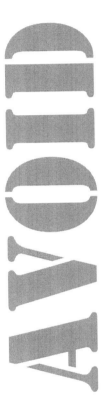

Herbs, Spices and Seasonings
Dark chocolate (72%+)
Raw honey
Sugar (brown and unrefined)

Beverages
Water (from the tap)
Wine (red or dry white — for best results, you should completely abstain from alcohol)

Sizedrop 42 Days to a New You Food Plan: Days 28-42

All You Can Eat

On days 28 to 42, you are **allowed to eat all** of the following foods listed. There's **no counting calories**, so simply choose from the list to satiate your appetite.

As always, buy organic whenever possible.

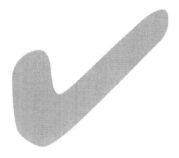

Meat and Poultry
Chicken
Duck
Goat
Goose
Pheasant
Quail
Rabbit
Turkey
Venison

Fish and Seafood
Herring/Kipper
Wild Salmon
Sardine
Snapper
Wild Trout

Nuts and Seeds
Almonds
Brazil nuts
Cashew nuts
Chestnuts
Hazelnuts
Macadamia nuts
Pecans
Pinenuts
Pistachio nuts
Poppy seeds
Pumpkin seeds
Sesame seeds
Sunflower seeds
Walnuts

As a Thank You for reading this book, please visit www.feellikeshit.co.uk for your FREE BOOK BONUS

Fruit

Apples
Apricots
Blackberries
Blueberries
Cherries
Coconut
Cranberries
Grapefruit
Kiwi
Lemon/Lime
Papaya
Pear
Plum
Pomegranate
Raspberries
Watermelon

Vegetables and Legumes

Aduki beans
Artichokes (globe and Jerusalem)
Asparagus
Aubergine
Avocado
Beet greens
Beetroot
Berlotti beans
Black beans
Black-eyed beans
Bok choy
Broad beans
Broccoli
Brussel sprouts
Butter beans
Butternut squash
Cabbage
Capers

As a Thank You for reading this book, please visit www.feellikeshit.co.uk for your FREE BOOK BONUS

Feel Like S**t?

Carrots
Cauliflower
Celeriac
Celery
Chard
Chickpeas
Courgette
Cucumber
Fennel
Garlic
Ginger
Green beans
Green peas
Kale
Kidney beans
Leeks
Lentils
Lettuce (iceberg/romaine)
Mangetout
Okra
Olives
Onions
Parsnips
Peppers
Pumpkin
Radish
Radicchio
Rocket
Spinach
Spring greens
Sprouts (aduki, alfalfa, lentil)
Squash
Suede
Sweet potato
Swiss chard
Tomatoes
Watercress

As a Thank You for reading this book, please visit www.feellikeshit.co.uk for your FREE BOOK BONUS

Dairy
Eggs
Goat whey

Oils and Fats
Butter (unsalted)
Coconut butter/oil
Flax or Hemp seed oil
Palm oil (sustainable)
Sesame oil
Extra virgin olive oil
Ghee

Herbs, Spices and Seasonings
Basil
Bay
Cardamon
Carob
Cayenne
Chilli
Chives
Cinnamon
Cloves
Coriander
Cumin
Curry powder
Dill
Fennel
Horseradish
Lemongrass
Mint
Mustard
Nutmeg
Oregano
Paprika
Parsley
Peppercorns

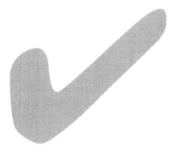

Feel Like S**t?

Peppermint
Rosemary
Sage
Sea salt
Turmeric
Vinegar (apple cider/balsamic)

Beverages

Almond milk
Coconut milk
Coconut water
Green tea
Herbal teas
Vegetable juices (unpasteurised)
Water (filtered or bottled)

Days 28-42

Menu suggestions

Breakfast
Poached egg with spinach and grilled tomatoes
Berry and banana smoothie
Wild smoked salmon with scrambled eggs
Poached egg and spinach on sourdough rye bread
Hot quinoa cereal with apple and cinnamon
Fruit, nuts and yogurt with coconut chips

Lunch
Kitcheri (see recipe on page 229)
Roast duck breast with salad of avocado, tomato and Roquefort
Baked wild trout with steamed greens

Dinner
Roast garlic and tarragon chicken with salad
Moroccan lamb and bean tagine
Homemade spicy meatballs with brown basmati rice
(see recipe on page 226)
Pan-fried mackerel with steamed broccoli
Thai green chicken curry (see recipe on page 227)

Snacks
Boiled egg and cucumber sticks
Rollmop herring and rice cakes
Avocado and goats cheese
Green vegetable juice
Nuts, seeds and coconut chips

Recipes

Juicy milks and juices

It is definitely worth investing in a juicer as part of your new healthier lifestyle. First, it is a great way to start the day as you mean to go on. In addition, it's a very easy way of making sure you get lots of nutrition in just one glass of juice. However, if you feel a juicer is too much of an expense at the moment, then don't worry, because almost everyone has access to a blender (or, alternatively, a hand blender), so you could easily make a nutritious smoothie instead.

Please buy organic or biodynamic fruits and vegetables whenever possible, as this is the only way you'll be able to protect yourself from any added pesticides and other harmful chemicals. For more details on pesticide levels in conventional and organic food, there's a great reference provided by the Environment Working Group in its Dirty Dozen and Clean 15, which you can find at www.ewg.org/foodnews/summary.

Cucumber, Kale, Apple and Lemon Juice

(Allowed on days 1-42)
Serves: 2

Ingredients:
1 large cucumber
1 large handful of kale
4 medium apples
1 lemon

Directions:
Juice all ingredients and drink immediately. Add a spoonful each of spirulina and chlorella for an optional immune system boost.

Celery, Pear, Spinach and Ginger Juice

(Allowed days 28-42)
Serves: 2

Ingredients:
6 stalks of celery
3 large pears
2 large handfuls of spinach
Thumb-sized piece of ginger

Directions:
Add all ingredients to a juicer and drink immediately. Added extras: add a teaspoonful of chia seeds to thicken juice.

Almond milk

(Allowed days 1-42)
Serves: 4

Ingredients:
1 cup almonds, soaked overnight and peeled
2 dates, soaked overnight in filtered water
1 litre filtered water
Optional: 1tsp cinnamon

Directions:
Combine all ingredients in a blender (or Vitamix), including the soak water from the dates, and process on high. Filter the liquid through a sieve or muslin cloth before serving in glasses or decanting into a wide-mouthed glass bottle. Drink your almond milk immediately, use it in a recipe, add it to your morning porridge... the choice is yours. It will keep for up to three days in the fridge.

Green Hydration Thick Smoothie

(Allowed days 28-42)
Serves: 1

I got home hungry one late afternoon, but I was too tired to cook a meal, nor did I fancy eating a salad. I also needed hydration, since I had been running around all day and hadn't drunk enough water. So I looked at what I had in the fridge and combined it into this smoothie — which is actually more like a 'thickie' and probably best drunk through a straw. Highly nutritious, it's kind of like a meal in a glass.

Ingredients:
300ml coconut water
100g fresh pineapple
100g fresh coconut
1tbsp of chia seeds
1tsp of chlorella
Large handful of spinach

Directions:
Combine all ingredients in a blender (or use a hand blender), then serve in a glass with a straw.

Easy lunches, dinners and sides

I believe that once you feel confident in the kitchen, cooking for yourself, and perhaps your family, will be an activity that you'll come to enjoy, rather than feeling like a chore. A good kitchen knife and cutting board is essential kit. There are many videos on YouTube that show how you can perfect your knife skills.

Luckily, the following recipes don't need the skills of a chef to make, nor do they take that much time to prepare. And they're all delicious and packed with loads of nutrition to help feed your body.

Spicy Sweet Potato Chips

(Allowed days 1-42)
Serves: 4

Ingredients:
6 sweet potatoes, peeled and cut into chunks
2tbsp coconut oil
Sea salt and freshly ground black pepper (*to taste*)
½ tsp cayenne pepper (*optional*)

Directions:
Preheat oven to 220°C. Mix ingredients together by hand in a large bowl, covering the potato chunks. Spread the chips out in a single layer on a large pre-heated baking tray.

Bake for about 15 minutes, or until crispy and brown on one side. Turn over and cook for another 10 minutes, or until they're crispy on the outside and tender inside. Cooking time will vary depending on how thick you cut your chips.

Kale and Avocado Salad

(Allowed days 1-42)
Serves: 2 (or 3 as a side dish)

Ingredients:
100g baby spinach and/or rocket leaves
2 large handfuls of kale, stalks removed and finely chopped
1 lime, juiced
1 large avocado, chopped into chunky pieces
1 spring onion, finely chopped
½ cucumber, peeled and chopped
Handful of sundried tomatoes, soaked if needed
Big handful of cherry tomatoes, sliced into half pieces
50g fresh pitted black olives (*not in brine*)
½ cup sprouts, such as alfalfa, broccoli, radish, mung, aduki (*on their own or in combinations*)
1tsp sea salt
Extra virgin olive oil

For the dressing:
10ml apple cider vinegar
10ml extra virgin olive oil
2 garlic cloves, very finely chopped
1tsp wholegrain mustard with seeds
Put all ingredients into a lidded glass jar. Tighten the lid and shake until the mustard dissolves.

Directions:
In a large bowl, marinate the kale by drizzling in olive oil and adding 1tsp of sea salt. Next, knead the kale with your fingers until the oil and salt have penetrated the leaves. If possible, cover and leave to sit for up to one hour.

In a small bowl, marinate the avocado and spring onion in the lime juice and the rest of the sea salt. Allow to sit for 10-15 minutes. Finally, add the remaining ingredients to the kale, combine, then fold in the avocado mixture. Pour over the dressing, toss and serve.

Quinoa, Broccoli and Egg Salad

(Allowed days 28-42)
Serves: 2

Ingredients:
A combination of baby greens, rocket and/or romaine lettuce
1 courgette, sliced into matchsticks
1 large chopped tomato,
1 small beet, shredded
1 boiled egg, chopped
1 head of steamed broccoli florets
2tbsp of nutritional yeast
½ cup cooked quinoa
Optional: poached salmon steak, flaked

Directions:
Combine all ingredients in a large bowl. Add a drizzle of extra virgin olive oil and balsamic or apple cider vinegar for a delicious and nutritious meal.

Boiled Eggs with Rye Toast and Radish Butter

(Allowed days 28-42)
Serves: 2

Ingredients:
50g grass-fed butter, softened
6 French breakfast radishes
4 slices of rye bread
4 medium organic eggs (*at room temperature*)
Sea salt and black pepper to taste

Directions:
Grate the radishes with a fine grater and place in a bowl lined with kitchen towel to absorb any extra moisture. Whip the butter with a fork until it's

very soft, then add the grated radishes and combine well. Season with sea salt and black pepper.

Bring a pan of water to a boil, add the eggs and simmer for three minutes. Turn off the heat, cover with a lid and leave to stand for two minutes. Meanwhile, toast the bread and spread with the radish butter. Cut slices into soldiers and serve with the soft-boiled egg.

Spicy Meatballs with Raita

(Allowed days 8-42)
Serves: 2

Tip: Make a large enough batch of meatballs for snacking and keep any leftovers in the fridge.

Ingredients:
For the meatballs:
250g organic lamb or beef mince
1tbsp ground coriander seeds
1tsp ground cumin powder
½ tsp cayenne pepper (depending on how spicy you like it!)
½ tsp cinnamon powder
1tbsp tomato puree
½ tsp black pepper
1tsp dried oregano or thyme
1tbsp ghee for frying
For the raita:
1 seedless cucumber, peeled and diced
1tsp salt
½ pot sheep or goat yogurt
1 spring onion, trimmed and thinly sliced
1tbsp fresh mint
Lemon juice to taste

Directions:
Place the cucumbers in a colander. Sprinkle with salt and let them sit in the sink for 15 minutes to drain. Rinse under cold water and drain again.

Feel Like S**t?

Combine the cucumber, yogurt, green onions, mint and lemon juice to taste. Cover and refrigerate for at least 30 minutes, then check seasoning, adding more salt and/or lemon juice, if necessary.

For the meatballs, blend all the ingredients (apart from the ghee) together in a bowl with the back of a fork. If the mixture remains very stiff, add a bit more tomato puree. Work the mixture into small balls in the palm of your hand and set aside — you should get about 6-8 meatballs. Heat the ghee and in a frying pan, gently fry the balls over a medium heat, turning occasionally. It should take about 10-15 minutes to brown them.

Serve with brown basmati rice and pour the raita on top. Sprinkle with a handful of lightly toasted almonds or cashew nuts. Delicious when served with a green salad.

Thai Green Chicken Curry

(Allowed days 28-42)
Serves: 4

Ingredients:
2tbsp coconut oil
Salt and freshly ground black pepper, for seasoning
1kg chicken thigh meat, skinned, boned and halved if large
2 onions, roughly chopped
2 sticks lemongrass, trimmed and finely chopped
4 cloves garlic, crushed
30g galangal or root ginger, scraped and finely chopped
1tbsp Thai green curry paste (*see recipe below*)
4 lime leaves
1.5ltr chicken stock
150ml coconut milk

Directions:
Heat the coconut oil in a heavy-bottomed saucepan, season the chicken thighs, place them in the pan and cook on a high heat for about 5 minutes.

227

Feel Like S**t?

Add the onions, lemongrass, garlic and galangal, and continue cooking for another 5 minutes.

Then add the curry paste (*see recipe below*), lime leaves and chicken stock. Bring to the boil, season and simmer for 40 minutes. Add the coconut milk and simmer for about another 10 minutes or until the sauce thickens. Serve with brown basmati rice.

Thai Green Curry Paste

Thai green curry paste is surprisingly easy to make, and it's so much healthier and tastes better than the store-bought variety. Added to your favourite meats, seafood or vegetables, this paste will create sumptuous curries. Or use it as a base to make delicious soups or noodle dishes. Cook with the paste straight away, or store in the refrigerator for up to two weeks. It can also be frozen for future use.

Ingredients:
1 stalk of lemongrass, minced
1-3 Thai green chilies, sliced
1 shallot, sliced, or 4 tbsp purple onion, minced
4-5 cloves garlic, minced
1 thumb-size piece of galangal or ginger, thinly sliced
Handful chopped fresh coriander/cilantro leaves and stems
Handful fresh Thai basil
½ tsp ground cumin
½ tsp Thai ground white pepper
½ tsp ground coriander
3tbsp fish sauce (*vegetarians: substitute ½tsp sea salt*)
½ tsp sea salt
2tbsp lime juice
3-4tbsp coconut milk (*enough to blend ingredients together*)

Directions:
Place all ingredients in a food processor, chopper or blender. Process well to form a paste. Test for seasoning — if too salty, add a squeeze of fresh lime or lemon, or more chilli for heat.

Feel Like S**t?

Tip: If using a pestle and mortar, pound all dry herbs and spices together to form a paste, and then gradually add all the wet ingredients, stirring until smooth.

Kitchari

(Allowed days 28-42)
Serves: 2
Whether you're looking to clean up your digestive system after years of abuse or just looking for a new tasty dish to add to your repertoire, cook up some kitchari for a complete food that will fill you up without weighing you down.

Ingredients:
Equal mix (about 1-2tbsp total) of seeds (cumin, fennel, fenugreek, coriander, mustard, nigella)
1tbsp curry powder
1tsp turmeric
1tbsp oil for sautéing (*I use raw virgin coconut oil*)
Equal parts (1 cup each) organic brown basmati rice and mung beans, both soaked in filtered water separately overnight
1 onion, chopped finely
2 crushed and chopped garlic cloves
1tsp minced ginger
1 cup root vegetable or squash cut in bite-sized pieces (sweet potato, pumpkin, butternut, onion squash, etc)
Hot water
Gomasio and toasted sesame oil to taste

Directions:
Drain soaked rice and mung beans. Boil a kettle. Gently fry seeds in a deep-lidded pan over medium heat until they start to pop. Add the onions, garlic and ginger until soft. Add the rice and mung beans, and stir to cover in the oil. Next, stir in the vegetables, then add the curry and turmeric, and stir. Now add enough hot water to more than cover the mixture so that the beans and rice have enough water to cook.

Feel Like S**t?

Cover with a lid and leave on low heat. Check every 5 minutes or so in case you need to add more water. It should be ready in about 20 minutes.

To serve, sprinkle with *gomasio* and toasted sesame oil, or serve with condiments of your choice. A favourite of mine is a dip made with sheep's yogurt, lime juice, grated raw garlic, finely chopped cucumber, mint and coriander, topped with pomegranate seeds. Yum!

Tip: If you can't find *gomasio*, you can make your own by crushing 2tbsp of lightly toasted sesame seeds and a large pinch of sea salt together in a pestle and mortar.

Sweet treats

To this day, I have to intentionally control my sugar intake and I've only accepted recently that I will always have a problem with sugar. But get this — I also came to the conclusion that everyone has a problem with sugar, because it's toxic and causes inflammation in the body.

Every time I consume too much sugar if I succumb to a slice of cake or normal dark chocolate bar, I bloat, feel uncomfortable and usually experience a lot of gas. These symptoms disappear after a couple of days away from the sweet death. Still, I'm only human and I can't but give in to treats every now and then. However, when I do, I try to keep them as clean as possible, and never do I consume anything containing high fructose corn syrup, glucose syrup or aspartame. Any sweet concoction containing any of these ingredients acts like poison in your body and will also play a part in making you even fatter.

The following treats will help to curb a sweet tooth while providing nutrition to the body.

Almond Butter

Almonds are full of antioxidants, which help to fight inflammation. Plus, in the form of almond butter, they taste delicious. Some almond butter spread on sprouted wheat bread is a great snack that can be used to satisfy a sweet craving, because the good fat in the almonds helps to fill you up. Have a clean jar ready to store your delicious nut butter.

Ingredients:
500g-1kg raw almonds

Directions:
Put all the almonds into a Magimix or food processor with a very powerful motor and turn on high speed. At first, the almonds will turn powdery and

231

flour-like. Continue processing and scraping the flour off the sides. Keep scraping down the sides for the next 5-7 minutes until the mixture turns dough-like, but do not stop the processing.

Your food processor may probably be quite warm at this point, so do be aware of this. After about another 3-5 minutes the doughy mixture will start to turn into a nut butter once all the oils become released.

Before decanting into a clean jar, you can mix in a pinch of fine pink Himalayan salt or drizzle of raw honey if desired.

Chocolate Avocado Pudding

(Allowed days 28-42)
Serves: 2-4

Ingredients:
2 avocados
¼ cup chopped dates
4tbsp raw cacao powder
2tbsp chopped nuts (walnuts, pecans, brazils and macadamias)

Directions:
In a high-speed blender, combine the avocado, dates and cacao powder, and blend together until smooth.

If your taste prefers, you may want to add up to 1tbsp water, depending on how thick you want your pudding.

Then fold in the chopped nuts and serve in small bowls. You can also garnish the pudding with fruit — bananas, strawberries, raspberries and cherries work particularly well — or top with a dollop of coconut cream. You can even use this pudding as 'icing' for cakes. It will keep in the fridge for up to three days.

Chocolate Chia Pudding

(Allowed days 28-42)
Serves: 1

Ingredients:
1 cup unsweetened almond or coconut milk
2tbsp chia seeds
1tsp raw cacao powder
½ tsp cinnamon
½ tbsp 100% pure maple syrup

Directions:
Combine all the ingredients into a large glass jar or container with a screw-top lid, then refrigerate for at least four hours, shaking at least once an hour to keep the seeds from sticking together.

To make extra servings, simply multiply the ingredients. It will keep for up to a week in the fridge. This pudding is delicious to eat on its own or topped with fresh fruit, toasted cashews or both.

Coconut Matcha Green Tea Smoothie

(Allowed days 1-42)
Serves: 1

Ingredients:
4tbsp fresh young coconut meat
½ banana
1 cup almond milk
2tsp Matcha green tea powder

Directions:
In a blender, combine all ingredients and blend together. Adjust proportions to taste and drink immediately.

233

Health benefits of some of the aforementioned foods

Apple cider vinegar (non-pasteurised and containing 'the mother') One tablespoon mixed in a glass of water, twice a day, has been known to promote weight loss in some individuals.

Almonds are packed with inflammation-fighting antioxidants, healthy plant fats and magnesium, which helps to regulate blood sugar levels and thus curbs emotional eating. Almonds also have the ability to lower bad LDL cholesterol, which aids in preventing coronary heart disease.

Apple juice (freshly juiced) provides beneficial antioxidants, as well as polyphenols, which help to regulate blood sugar levels.

Cacao is the purest form of chocolate and is actually good for you. Containing antioxidant flavonoids, sulfur and magnesium, the essential fatty acids found in cacao may help the body to regulate its good and bad cholesterol levels.

Celery juice is anti-inflammatory and helps to regulate any sweet cravings.

Chia seeds are packed full of omega 3s, proteins and antioxidants.

Chlorella helps the body break down toxic heavy metals such as mercury and lead, boosts the immune system and normalises blood pressure and blood sugar levels.

Coconut (fresh young) The meat from a young Thai coconut is a medium-chain saturated fat, but has many health benefits, including the fact that the liver quickly converts medium-chain triglycerides into energy.

Coconut oil is the only fat that can tolerate being heated at high temperatures without turning into trans fats. Processed coconut, such as desiccated, does not have the same health benefits.

As a Thank You for reading this book, please visit www.feellikeshit.co.uk for your FREE BOOK BONUS

Feel Like S**t?

Coconut water is packed full of electrolytes and B complex vitamins, plus research shows its cytokinins (plant hormones) have a significant anti-aging effect on the body.

Cucumbers are a great source of B vitamins and help the body to eliminate toxins from the digestive system. Due to a low calorie and high water content, cucumbers are an ideal dietary addition for those looking to lose weight. Daily consumption is a remedy for chronic constipation. Cucumbers also contain potassium, magnesium and fibre, which work effectively at regulating blood pressure.

Ginger juice also contains antioxidant and anti-inflammatory properties.

Kale juice is considered the most nutritious vegetable juice because of its powerful antioxidant, anti-inflammatory and anti-cancer properties. It's also a great immune booster, is high in beta-carotene, vitamins C and K, lutein, zeaxanthin and calcium.
However, those individuals diagnosed with kidney, gallbladder or thyroid conditions should avoid consuming kale juice.

Lemons are not only high in vitamin C, but lemon juice is alkalising to the body, so helps to balance the body's pH levels. It also contains calcium, magnesium and potassium, and is great for the skin.

Matcha green tea contains a group of catechin antioxidants known as EGCGs, which help to reduce inflammation, as well as speed up metabolism to aid weight loss. Matcha also helps to curb the appetite and contains L-theanine, an amino acid that causes the mind to calm, thus promoting relaxation.

Mung beans are a staple of the cleansing Ayurvedic diet and a perfect food for helping aid weight loss. They're a rich source of protein and fibre, which helps aid digestion, and are also effective in helping to keep blood sugar levels balanced.

Nutritional yeast is a rich source of protein and vitamins, including one of the few non-animal sources of B12, much missing in most vegetarian and vegan diets. It is also rich in amino and folic acids, iron, magnesium, phosphorus, zinc, chromium and selenium.

As a Thank You for reading this book, please visit www.feellikeshit.co.uk for your FREE BOOK BONUS

Feel Like S**t?

Pear juice is also anti-inflammatory and helps to keep your bowels regular.

Pineapple juice provides almost all the vitamins and minerals essential for a healthy digestive tract. Fresh pineapple juice stimulates the kidneys, relieves intestinal disorders and has diuretic properties. Along with many other benefits, fresh raw pineapple juice reduces excess fluid build-up in the cells.

Spinach juice is loaded with iron, calcium, vitamins E, C, A, B9, K and other vital nutrients that are needed for keeping the body healthy.

Spirulina is a blue-green algae grown in freshwater that can help boost your immune system, regulate cholesterol and high blood pressure, and is rich in protein.

Sprouts (alfalfa, mung, aduki, broccoli, china rose, radish, chickpea, lentil) are highly nutritious and contain a greater concentration of vitamins, minerals, proteins, enzymes, phytochemicals, antioxidants, trace mineral and bioflavonoids than at any other point in a plant's life.

The abundant enzymes contained in sprouts makes them easily digestible. An alkalising food, they can be eaten on their own in salads, added at the end of a stir-fry or juiced in a green drink.

Turmeric contains curcumin, which is a natural antiseptic and anti-bacterial agent with anti-inflammatory properties that has been shown to slow down the growth of certain cancers. It may also aid in the body's fat metabolism and help in the management of weight loss.

Best and Worst List

This is a general list you can use to remind yourself of the best and worst options you have available when eating fats, sugars and grains. Remember also that the consumption of too much sugar will cause inflammation — even after your detoxification. By all means you can use it, simply be aware of any effects that you may have after consuming too much and how that makes your body feel.

FATS
Good
Coconut oil (*for cooking/baking*)
Extra virgin olive oil (*for salad dressing*)
Butter (*organic or grass-fed only*)
Ghee (*organic or grass-fed only*)
Nuts and seeds
Avocado
Young green coconut meat

Bad
Low-fat
Trans-fat
Rapeseed/Canola oil
Hydrogenated oil
Vegetable oil
Margarine

GRAINS
Good
Quinoa
Spelt
Barley
Amaranth
Wholewheat pasta (*in moderation*)
Whole brown rice
Rye bread (*in moderation*)
Spelt bread (*in moderation*)
Sprouted bread (*health food shops*)

Bad
White bread
White pasta
White rice

SUGARS

Good (but used sparingly)

Raw or manuka honey
100% pure maple syrup
Stevia (*leaf or liquid tincture only; the white crystal variety readily available is processed*)
100% pure date syrup
Coconut palm sugar
Organic Blackstrap molasses
Dark (or raw) chocolate, at least a 72% cacao

Bad

High fructose corn syrup
Corn syrup
Cane juice
Glucose-fructose syrup
Fructose
Sucrose
Glucose
Dextrose
Maltose
Maltodextrin
Malt syrup
Rice syrup
Cane sugar
White sugar
Icing sugar
Golden syrup
Fruit juice concentrate
White and milk chocolate

Natural Health Resources

HEALTH FOOD AND NEWS WEBSITES

www.localfoods.org.uk
www.foodmatters.tv
www.ewg.org
www.mercola.com
www.naturalsociety.com
www.naturalnews.com
www.pollyspath.com
www.kriscarr.com
www.mindbodygreen.com
www.globalhealingcenter.com
www.detoxyourworld.com
www.therawfoodcoach.com
www.juicemaster.com
www.local-farmers-markets.co.uk
www.lfm.org.uk
www.bigbarn.co.uk
www.hookandson.co.uk
www.localfoodadvisor.com

BOOKS

The China Study T Colin Campbell, Thomas M Campbell II
Healing With Wholefoods: Asian Traditions and Modern Nutrition
Paul Pitchford
Pure, White and Deadly: How Sugar Is Killing Us and What We Can Do To Stop It John Yudkin and Robert H Lustig MD
Fat Chance: Beating the Odds Against Sugar, Processed Food, Obesity and Disease Robert H Lustig MD
Hungry For Change James Colquhoun, Laurentine ten Bosch, Mark Hyman
Why We Get Fat: And What to Do About It Gary Taubes

FILMS
Food Inc, 2008
Fat, Sick & Nearly Dead, 2010
King Corn: You Are What You Eat, 2007
Hungry For Change, 2012
Foodmatters, 2009
Forks Over Knives, 2011
Crazy Sexy Cancer, 2008
The Weight of the Nation, Episode 101 "Poverty and Obesity: When Healthy Food Isn't an Option", 2012
Fast Food Nation, 2006
Supersize Me, 2004
Fresh, 2009
Sicko, 2007
May I Be Frank, 2010
Killer At Large, 2008

CHEMICAL-FREE PERSONAL CARE PRODUCTS AND COSMETICS
www.ewg.org/skindeep (*database of harmful chemicals in cosmetics*)
www.lovelula.com
www.theorganicpharmacy.com
www.greenpeople.co.uk
www.biggreensmile.com
www.thedailygreen.com
www.soorganic.com
www.bentleyorganic.com
www.mypure.co.uk
www.fushi.co.uk
www.naturisimo.com
www.lilylolo.co.uk
www.suvarna.co.uk
www.essential-care.co.uk

As a Thank You for reading this book, please visit www.feellikeshit.co.uk for your FREE BOOK BONUS

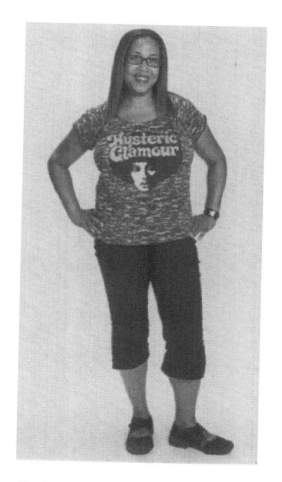

Here I am at a UK size 20 — the big smile is because this
picture was taken the day before I decided to begin my first detox.
Photo courtesy of *Black Beauty and Hair*

As a Thank You for reading this book, please visit www.feellikeshit.co.uk for your
FREE BOOK BONUS

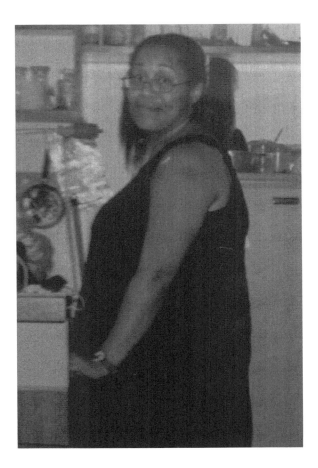

This was my favourite dress at the time, because it hid a multitude of fat.
And no, I'm not pregnant in this picture, as some have questioned.

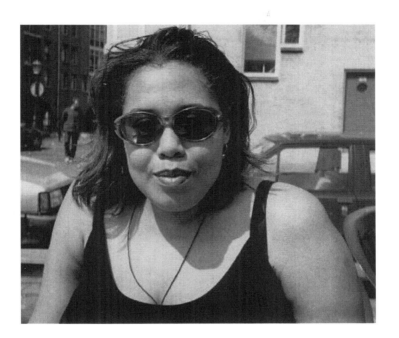

Bloated, uncomfortable and forcing a smile.

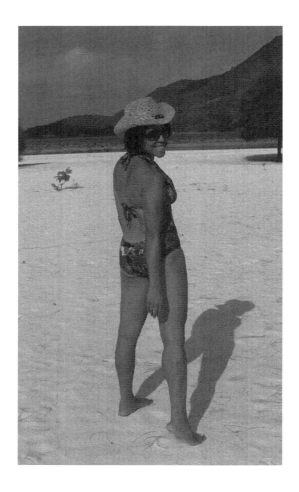

Feeling good on the beach, having dropped 75lbs.

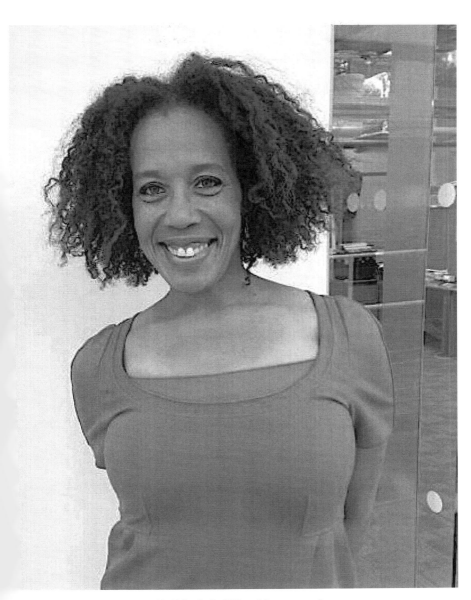

At 49, I don't feel like shit anymore!

As a Thank You for reading this book, please visit www.feellikeshit.co.uk for your FREE BOOK BONUS

ATTENTION, ALL YO-YO AND FED-UP FAD DIETERS AND BINGE EATERS!
It's Time To Break This Vicious Cycle...

BY JOINING ME AT:

www.feellikeshit.co.uk/members/book

where you'll get a FREE

30-day trial membership*, as well as access to:

<u>THE EVILS OF ASPARTAME</u>
TELESEMINAR

An in-depth look at how artificial sugar is the real slimmer's enemy... including:

- *Why aspartame is toxic*

- *Why food manufacturers are allowed to use it*

- *How aspartame makes you fat*

- *The science behind the poison*